"We have learned so much about the viral pandemic's social and psychological consequences in the major global research hubs, but we do not know much about how the countries in the peripheries of these hubs have experienced and responded to the pandemic. In *COVID-19 and Psychology in Malaysia: Psychosocial Effects, Coping, and Resilience,* we are provided a thoughtful entry point for exploring the socio-psychological experiences of Malaysians during the pandemic. The various chapters provide snapshots in different domains of Malaysia society that point to some convergences with universal pandemic experiences and to how some specific sociocultural practices characterize aspects of Malaysian's COVID-19 pandemic experiences. There is so much to learn from this volume."

Professor Allan B. Bernardo,
Distinguished University Professor and University Fellow,
De La Salle University Manila,
Former President, ASEAN Regional Union of Psychological Societies

COVID-19 and Psychology in Malaysia

Part of a mini series of Focus books on COVID-19 in Malaysia, the chapters in this book address the psychosocial impact on the pandemic and ways in which people have learned to develop the ability to be more resilient despite the challenges of living and working during this public health crisis.

Covering a range of topics including life under lockdown, working on the frontlines, and the rapid adaptation to online teaching, the contributors highlight the pervasiveness of the pandemic on Malaysian society, identified factors that potentially increase the psychosocial impact of the pandemic on different segments of the population and how Malaysians have found ways to cope throughout this period. This is an opportunity to witness how researchers from multiple disciplines can join forces during challenging times. There are a great many lessons to be learned from the successes and failures in responding to the pandemic and the measures that have been necessary to contain it.

A fascinating read for scholars with an interest in crisis management in non-Western contexts, especially those with a particular interest in Malaysia, or Southeast Asia more generally.

D. Gerard Joseph Louis (The chief editor of the psychology book) is the Pro Vice-Chancellor (Mental Health), Dean of the Faculty of Behavioral Sciences, Education and Languages at HELP University, Kuala Lumpur and the CEO of the HELP Education Services, a subsidary of the HELP International Corporation that oversees the management of the K-12 International Schools Division. He has been involved in the field of education, counselling and training for over 30 years.

Gerard is a Counselling Psychologist and has extensive experience in the supervision and development of both professional counsellors and counsellors-in-training. His research and professional interests are in the areas of resilience and well-being. Over the period of the Movement Control Order (MCO) from March to July, 2020, he was involved in offering webinars to private and government organisations and the public at large on issues related to managing mental health and well-being during periods of uncertainty brought about by COVID-19 pandemic. He also led the initiatives of the Department of Psychology at HELP in the delivery of a host of virtual events, podcasts and other resources in response to the mental health issues arising from the pandemic (https://university.help.edu.my/mental-health-response-to-COVID-19/)

Surinderpal Kaur (The editor of *COVID-19 in Malaysia* multidisciplinary series) is an Associate Professor and Dean at the Faculty of Languages and Linguistics, Universiti Malaya, Malaysia. She attained her PhD from Lancaster University, UK. Her research interests include Media Discourses and Multimodality, focusing specifically upon public discourses in mainstream and social media that relate to public health, migration, and terrorism issues. She has been actively involved with Universiti Malaya's social outreach initiatives to offer solutions to the mental health challenges faced by Malaysian during the COVID-19 pandemic (Caring Together/UMPrihatin), focusing specifically on the social media platforms Telegram and Facebook. She is currently compiling a database of research and data from all over the world to help Malaysian scholars in their research on COVID-19.

Huey Fen Cheong (The managing editor of *COVID-19 in Malaysia* multidisciplinary series) is a Senior Lecturer in the Department of English Language, Faculty of Languages and Linguistics, Universiti Malaya. Her research interests are interdisciplinary from gender studies and linguistics to marketing and psychology. Her works are usually humanitarian, from gender equality (for men and women) and anti-racism (skin whitening and Black Lives Matter) to decolonisation of academia. The last one explains the initiative behind this book series in creating a platform for researchers to study the COVID-19 pandemic in Malaysia, which addresses the lack of COVID-19 research and publication in South East Asia. She is also the founder of the Facebook group, (Post-)COVID job market in Malaysia (https://www.facebook.com/groups/2805574166392321), which shares information about the new normal of employment and employability during this challenging time.

COVID-19 in Asia

COVID-19, Business, and Economy in Malaysia
Retrospective and Prospective Perspectives
Edited by Weng Marc Lim, Surinderpal Kaur, and Huey Fen Cheong

COVID-19, Education, and Literacy in Malaysia
Social Contexts of Teaching and Learning
Edited by Ambigapathy Pandian, Surinderpal Kaur, and Huey Fen Cheong

COVID-19 and Psychology in Malaysia
Psychosocial Effects, Coping, and Resilience
Edited by D. Gerard Joseph Louis, Surinderpal Kaur, and Huey Fen Cheong

COVID-19 and Psychology in Malaysia

Psychosocial Effects, Coping, and Resilience

Edited by D. Gerard Joseph Louis, Surinderpal Kaur, and Huey Fen Cheong

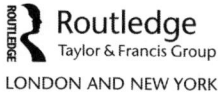
Routledge
Taylor & Francis Group

LONDON AND NEW YORK

First published 2022
by Routledge
2 Park Square, Milton Park, Abingdon, Oxon OX14 4RN

and by Routledge
605 Third Avenue, New York, NY 10158

Routledge is an imprint of the Taylor & Francis Group, an Informa business

British Library Cataloguing-in-Publication Data
A catalogue record for this book is available from the British Library

Library of Congress Cataloguing-in-Publication Data
Names: Louis, D. Gerard Joseph, editor. | Kaur, Surinderpal,
    editor. | Fen Cheong, Huey, editor.
Title: COVID-19 and psychology in Malaysia: psychosocial effects,
    coping and resilience/edited by D. Gerard Joseph Louis,
    Surinderpal Kaur and Huey Fen Cheong.
Description: Milton Park, Abingdon, Oxon; New York, NY:
    Routledge, 2022.
Identifiers: LCCN 2021031701 (print) | LCCN 2021031702
    (ebook) | ISBN 9781032014241 (hardback) | ISBN
    9781032014258 (paperback) | ISBN 9781003178576 (ebook)
Subjects: LCSH: COVID-19 (Disease)–Malaysia. | COVID-19
    (Disease)–Psychological aspects–Malaysia. | COVID-19 Pandemic,
    2020–Malaysia.
Classification: LCC RA644.C67 C68319 2022 (print) |
    LCC RA644.C67 (ebook) | DDC 362.1962/414009595–dc23
LC record available at https://lccn.loc.gov/2021031701
LC ebook record available at https://lccn.loc.gov/2021031702

ISBN: 978-1-032-01424-1 (hbk)
ISBN: 978-1-032-01425-8 (pbk)
ISBN: 978-1-003-17857-6 (ebk)

DOI: 10.4324/9781003178576

Typeset in Galliard
by KnowledgeWorks Global Ltd.

Contents

List of figures   xi
List of tables   xii
List of contributors   xiv
Preface   xix
Acknowledgements   xxiii

SECTION I
Working during the pandemic   1

1 Psychological distress among healthcare professionals
   at the frontlines: Anaesthesiologists' perspective   3
   SAMUEL ERN HUNG TSAN, ANAND KAMALANATHAN, & CHEW YIN WANG

2 Psychological distress among essential and non-essential
   service workers   19
   MARC ARCHER & CHEE HOONG MOEY

SECTION II
Predictors of distress and mental health   37

3 Psychosocial and demographic predictors of mental
   health and distress   39
   HASSE DE MEYER, FARIHIN UFIYA, & SIEW LI NG

4 Women's emotional health and support in a time of crisis   54
   VIMALA BALAKRISHNAN, KEE SEONG NG, & AZMAWATY MOHAMAD NOR

SECTION III
Developing resilience during the pandemic   71

5 Psychological impact and the use of religious coping among
   Malaysian Catholic older adults   73
   D. GERARD JOSEPH LOUIS, CLARENCE DEVADASS, PAULINE
   POOI YIN LEONG, MELISSA SHAMINI PERRY, & YUEN BENG LEE

6 Factors promoting university instructor's resilience
   to technostress   89
   CHIA KEAT YAP & SI NA KEW

7 The relationship between emotion regulation and
   well-being during the pandemic: Resilience as a mediator   104
   NURUL IZZAH FATHIAH BINTI WAN ALI MUNAWAR & EUGENE Y. J. TEE

List of figures

1.1 Factors associated with anaesthesiologists' burnout and
depression risk: (a) burnout vs. depression risk
($p < 0.0001$); (b) number of calls vs. depression risk
($p = 0.026$) and (c) number of calls vs. burnout ($p = 0.038$)   11

1.2 Association between anaesthesiologists' worry of
COVID-19 with (a) burnout ($p = 0.014$) and
(b) depression risk ($p = 0.044$)   11

4.1 Depression and stress prevalence rates based on
their severity levels   61

6.1 The evaluation of measurement model using PLS-SEM   95

7.1 Path plot of the significant indirect effect of reappraisal
on well-being through resilience   113

List of tables

1.1 Respondents' (anaesthesiologists') characteristics ($n = 85$) 8

1.2 Burnout, depression risk, worry about COVID-19 and medical errors among respondents ($n = 85$) 9

1.3 Multivariate logistic regression analysis for burnout and depression risk 12

2.1 Severity categories of depression and anxiety symptoms for total sample, and essential versus non-essential service subgroups with comparison of proportion above clinical cut-off 25

2.2 Service area for essential service workers ($n = 73$) and job category non-essential service workers ($n = 104$) 26

2.3 Scores of depression and anxiety for total sample and subgroups 26

2.4 Correlations between Behaviours and Concerns Amidst Pandemic Scale (BCAPS) variables and indicators of psychological distress scores (PHQ-9 for depression and GAD-7 for anxiety) ($n = 173$) 28

2.5 Summary of log-linked gamma generalised linear model for BCAPS variables predicting psychological distress scores (PHQ-9 for depression and GAD-7 for anxiety) ($n = 173$) 29

3.1 Demographic characteristics of respondents (Malaysian residents) ($n = 1,234$) 44

3.2 Prevalence of mental distress and its associated odd ratio by predictor category 48

4.1 Demographics of the women respondents 60

4.2 Binary logistic regressions for emotional distress 62

4.3 Descriptive statistics for emotional support 62

4.4 Linear regression for emotional support 63

5.1 General description of interview respondents (Catholic
older adults) 78
6.1 Demographic profile of respondents (university instructors) 93
6.2 Convergent validity of measurement model in PLS-SEM 96
6.3 Discriminant validity (HTMT ratio) of measurement
model in PLS-SEM 96
6.4 Results of hypothesis testing using PLS-SEM 97
7.1 Bivariate correlation table for reappraisal, suppression,
resilience and well-being 112
7.2 Tests of hypothesised mediating effects of resilience
on the relationships between reappraisal and well-being,
and between suppression and well-being 113

List of contributors

Marc Archer has directed the Centre for Mental Health and Wellbeing—a collaboration between HELP University and the Malaysian Mental Health Association—since its founding in 2020.He has a background in social emotional developmental research and has studied the impact of separation from family on child and adolescent development in the US, UK, China and Malaysia. He has also been involved in several projects to increase access to mental health services, particularly among those less likely to seek help. His current work builds on this to adapt, implement and evaluate culture-specific interventions to enhance mental health and well-being.

Vimala Balakrishnan is an Associate Professor, affiliated with the Faculty of Computer Science and Information Technology, Universiti Malaya. Dr Balakrishnan's main research interests are in data analytics and sentiment analysis, particularly related to social media. She has published approximately 60 articles in top indexed journals and 45 conference proceedings. She has received several prestigious awards, including the Leadership in Innovation Fellowship (by the Royal Academy of Engineering, UK), and the Fulbright Scholar Award 2018. Dr Balakrishnan was recently listed as one of the top 2% world scientists by the Stanford University, 2020.

Hasse de Meyer is a licensed Clinical Psychologist and Senior Lecturer in the Master of Clinical Psychology program at HELP University, Malaysia. She completed her doctoral degree in Clinical Psychology at KU Leuven, Belgium. Her research focuses on reinforcement learning and developmental disorders in children and adolescents. Her key expertise is in Attention Deficit Hyperactivity Disorder, in which she has published in international peer-reviewed journals.

Clarence Devadass is a Catholic Priest and the Director of the Catholic Research Centre, Malaysia. As a Visiting Research Associate with the University of Nottingham Malaysia and a former Visiting Fellow at the Faculty of Divinity, University of Cambridge, UK, he continues to teach, write and speak at various platforms.

Anand Kamalanathan graduated with a Master of Anaesthesia (M.Anaes) in 2018 and subsequently served as an anaesthesiologist in Hospital Sungai Buloh, Selangor, from 2018 to 2021. He was actively involved in the management of critically ill COVID-19 patients in the ICU. He is currently pursuing his subspeciality as a Clinical Fellow in Cardiothoracic Anaesthesia at the National Heart Institute, Kuala Lumpur, Malaysia.

Si Na Kew is a Senior Lecturer at Language Academy, Faculty of Social Sciences and Humanities, Universiti Teknologi Malaysia. She received a bachelor in TESL at Universiti Teknologi Malaysia and completed her PhD studies in educational technology at Universiti Teknologi Malaysia. Her research interests are educational technology, online teaching and learning, learning analytics (LA), teaching English as a second language (TESL), technology enhanced language learning (TELL), computer assisted language learning (CALL), etc. She is currently one of the affiliates of the Young Scientist Network Academy of Sciences Malaysia (YSN-ASM). She is an editor of *Innovative Teaching and Learning Journal.*

Yuen Beng Lee is a Programme Leader and Senior Lecturer with the Department of Film and Performing Arts, School of Arts, Sunway University, Malaysia. He is co-editor of Democratic Transition and Political Change: Malaysia's Media at Election Crossroads. His research interests are in Malaysian cinema, media, communication and cultural studies.

Pauline Pooi Yin Leong is an Associate Professor with the Department of Communication, School of Arts, Sunway University, Malaysia. She is also a Research Fellow in Communication for the Christian Institute for Theological Engagement (CHRISTE). Her research interests are in political communication, digital media, freedom of speech and journalism.

D. Gerard Joseph Louis is one of the authors of Chapter 5 and the Chief Editor of this book. Please refer to the editor's biodata for more details.

Chee-Hoong Moey is a psychiatrist at the Department of Psychiatry and Mental Health, Selayang Hospital. He obtained his medical degree from International Medical University, Malaysia in February 2009 and Master in Psychological Medicine from Universiti Malaya in 2019. He is currently a committee member of the Early Career Psychiatrists (ECP)

Chapter of Malaysian Psychiatric Association. His areas of interest include consultation liaison psychiatry, neuropsychiatry and psychodynamic therapy.

Azmawaty Mohamad Nor is a Senior Lecturer in the Department of Educational Psychology and Counselling, Faculty of Education, Universiti Malaya, and a Registered Counsellor with the Board of Counsellors, Malaysia. She participated in the Tele-Health (Talian Kasih) helpline during the lockdown due to the COVID-19 pandemic. As an active researcher involved in numerous researches, she aspires to tap into the different areas thereby broadening her horizon and enhancing her quality of teaching and learning. Her areas of expertise include women studies, at-risks adolescence, substance abuse and work–life balance. She recently participated in three COVID-19–related studies.

Nurul Izzah Fathiah binti Wan Ali Munawar recently graduated with a Bachelor of Psychology (Hons.) from HELP University, where she now works as a graduate tutor at the Department of Psychology. She has research interests in the regulation of emotions, psychological resilience and well-being, and plans to pursue her Masters in Counselling at HELP University.

Kee Seong Ng received his PhD in Neurogastroenterology (2012) at Queen Mary, University of London. He is currently appointed as a Senior Medical Lecturer in Universiti Malaya.

Siew Li Ng completed her doctoral degree in Clinical Psychology from Central Michigan University (CMU), USA. She received specialized clinical trainings on anxiety, trauma-related and neuropsychological issues at CMU as well as on severe mental illness at University of Arizona, USA. She is currently a Senior Lecturer and the program chair for the Master's in Clinical Psychology program at HELP University. Her research focuses on addiction, trauma and anxiety issues. She also conducts psychotherapy and provides workshops for individual clients and organisations respectively on mental health concerns such as depression, anxiety, trauma and addiction.

Melissa Shamini Perry is a Senior Lecturer at the Centre for Research in Language and Linguistics, Faculty of Social Sciences and Humanities, National University of Malaysia. She is also a section editor for GEMA Online® *Journal of Language Studies* and a Research Fellow in Social Semiotics and Multimodality at the Christian Institute for Theological Engagement (CHRISTE). Her research interests are in the area of social semiotics, multimodality, applied literature, cultural narratives and alternative assessments.

Eugene Y.J. Tee is Associate Professor at the Department of Psychology, HELP University, Malaysia. He attained his PhD in Management from the University of Queensland in 2010 and has research interests in emotion-related processes in organisations and positive psychology. He has published work in *Leadership Quarterly, Asian Journal of Social Psychology,* and *Research on Emotions in Organizations.* Dr Tee is a Human Resource Development Fund (HRDF) Certified Trainer and has conducted emotions management training sessions for public and private sector organisations. He is a regular speaker on BFM89.9, and author of three books—the latest being *The Science of Feelings.*

Samuel Ern Hung Tsan is a Clinical Lecturer and Consultant Anaesthesiologist serving in the Universiti Malaysia Sarawak and Sarawak General Hospital, with a special interest in the field of neuroanaesthesiology and airway management. He completed his Master of Anaesthesiology (with distinction) from Universiti Malaya in 2020, and is a Fellow with the College of Anaesthesiologists of Ireland. A keen researcher, he is involved in numerous research projects, with multiple publications to his name. He also has a passion in teaching and has devoted himself to training the next generation of medical doctors.

Farihin Ufiya received her BSc in Psychology from HELP University, where she now works as a research assistant. She is also currently an officer to the Health Minister of Malaysia and the founding director of a mental health non-profit organisation. She is interested in the neural antecedents to voluntary action and will be pursuing her MSc in Neuroscience at University College London (UCL).

Chew Yin Wang is an Honorary Professor of the Department of Anaesthesiology, Faculty of Medicine, Universiti Malaya. She has published >80 papers, including co-authors in three papers in *N Engl J Med*, two in *Lancet* and three in *JAMA*. She has a highly successful collaboration with the Population Health Research Institute (PHRI), Canada, University of Toronto, Hong Kong University and Vita-Salute San Raffaele University, Italy making major contributions to POISE, POISE-2, POISE-3, VISION, VISION Cardiac Surgery, HIP-Attack, NeuroVision, MYRIAD Trial and POSA. She is currently Principal Investigator in Malaysia and Member Steering Committee for POISE-3 and COP-AF trials.

Chia Keat Yap is a Senior Lecturer and Programme Leader for Psychology at Asia Pacific University of Technology and Innovation (APU). He received his Master's degree in Abnormal and Clinical Psychology at Swansea University, Wales, United Kingdom and completed his PhD studies in Educational Psychology at University Technology Malaysia. His current research interests lie primarily in psychological resilience, all-but-dissertation (ABD), human-computer interaction and post-COVID-19 adaptation. He has more than 8 years of teaching experience in higher education institutions. He is also a reviewer for the *Universal Journal of Psychology*.

Preface

The World Health Organization (March 18, 2020) declared COVID-19 a global public health crisis. While a lot of the focus over the last year has been dealing with the physical health effects of the COVID-19 pandemic that has since ravaged communities globally, a more subtle but parallel mental health crisis, has also been developing. From educators and their students and retrenched workers to frontline medical workers and vulnerable members of the community (like the elderly or women), it is unsurprising to read reports of people from all walks of life experiencing feelings of fear and distress, arising from the new way of living and uncertainties brought about by COVID-19.

This book, entitled *"COVID-19 and Psychology in Malaysia: Psychosocial Effects, Coping, and Resilience"*, addresses the psychological impact of the COVID-19 pandemic in Malaysia. This book covers three key areas of focus, namely: (a) the experience of working during the pandemic, (b) predictors of mental health and distress and (c) developing resilience during the pandemic. Taken together, this book presents a composite picture of the psychosocial effects of the pandemic in Malaysia across a wide spectrum of everyday normal human activities. It also examines a range of factors that contribute towards mental health and elevated levels of distress in individuals and specific groups of people. Finally, it discusses factors that can help people cope with the uncertainties of this period and develop a higher level of resilience in times of distress and crisis. The chapters in this book present studies carried out between May 2020 to January 2021. They analysed the psychological impact during the various phases of the Movement Control Order (MCO), from the first MCO in March 2020 to the start of 2021. The MCO was enacted by the Malaysian Government to minimise social gatherings, in order to prevent the spread of the COVID-19 virus.

Section I, *Working during the pandemic*, features investigations of those working in essential and non-essential services in the early months of the pandemic and presents a snapshot of the prevalence and source of psychological distress of these workers during this period.

In Chapter 1, *Psychological distress among healthcare professionals at the frontlines—Anaesthesiologists' perspective,* Samuel Ern Hung Tsan from Universiti Malaysia Sarawak, Anand Kamalanathan from Sungai Buloh Hospital and Chew Yin Wang from Universiti Malaya discuss the prevalence of burnout and self-perceived medical errors committed by critical frontline healthcare professionals, specifically Anaesthesiologists, who worked at a designated COVID-19 hospital. While there were elevated levels of burnout, depression risks and medical errors committed during the period of assessment, burnout and depression risks were not significantly related to medical errors. They were, however, able to show that depression and burnout were significantly related to each other. The authors suggest that the high prevalence of psychological distress (i.e. burnout and depression risks) among critical frontline health workers indicates a parallel pandemic, which needs to be addressed, not only at the individual level, but also at the organisational, national and international levels, given that COVID-19 is a global pandemic. Recommendations for psychoeducational programmes for individuals to organisational support and community mental health programmes are discussed.

In Chapter 2, *Psychological distress among essential and non-essential service workers,* Marc Archer from HELP University and Chee Hoong Moey from Selayang Hospital, explore psychological distress (namely, the rates of depression and anxiety), among both essential and non-essential frontline workers in the early stages of the COVID-19 pandemic in Malaysia. Contrary to previous studies, this study showed that workers in both essential and non-essential services showed elevated levels of psychological distress across the workforce. The key reason for this is the uncertainty surrounding the progress of the pandemic. To mitigate this sense of uncertainty, the authors suggest the need for employers to be mindful of the role that uncertainty plays in psychological distress and to increase their efforts to strengthen processes in their operations, which provide as much certainty and stability as possible in their communications with their workers. Finally, specific pandemic-related concerns, such as close *contact with positive cases* and *the lack of time with family,* were shown to be linked to higher levels of anxiety, which should be noted, but with the latter requiring further investigation.

Section II, *Predictors of distress and mental health,* explores psychological and socio-demographic indicators, which may provide insights into why certain people in our population are more vulnerable to distress and mental health issues.

In Chapter 3, *Psychosocial and demographic predictors of mental health and distress*, Hasse De Meyer, Farihin Ufiya and Siew Li Ng—all of whom are from HELP University (with Hasse also affiliated with KU Leuven, Belgium)—investigate what aspects of Malaysia's unique demographic makeup and socioeconomic environment contribute towards mental health and distress during this particularly challenging period. Younger age, female, lower income (less than RM 2000), presence of a chronic illness and psychiatric history, and employment status were associated with poorer mental health outcomes. In addition, increased social media use, becoming unemployed, experiencing limited social support and feeling lonely were key factors that were associated with depressive and anxiety symptoms. The authors make a comparison of their findings with those of some western countries (e.g. Belgium, the United Kingdom and Italy) and highlight unique features in collectivist societies like Malaysia, which contribute towards lower mental health outcomes. Recommendations to improve mental health interventions, which are culturally sensitive, easily accessible and financially affordable, are discussed.

In Chapter 4, *Women's emotional health and support in a time of crisis*, Vimala Balakrishnan, Kee Seong Ng and Azmawaty Mohamad Nor, all of whom are from the Universiti Malaya, discuss the sociodemographic factors that predict both emotional distress and the need for emotional support among women. (*Note: Women are considered to be a particularly vulnerable group due to an increase in reports of gender-based violence during this pandemic period.*) The authors revealed that just over a third of their sample experienced some level of emotional distress, from mild to severe. Demographic factors, such as younger age (younger women) and decreased household income, are the key predictors of higher levels of distress. Women with lower income and lower level of education were also deemed to be in a greater need of social support from others. Interestingly, the majority of women in the study were found to be quite resilient, as they managed their distress on their own or with their family members only. Education was a key factor in explaining this outcome, as more than 90% of the women in this study had at least a university degree.

Section III, *Developing resilience during the pandemic*, highlights the mediating role of resilience in emotion regulation and well-being as well as identifies factors and coping strategies, which contribute to the development of resilience.

In Chapter 5, *Psychological impact and the use of religious coping among Malaysian Catholic older adults*, D. Gerard Joseph Louis from HELP University, Clarence Devadass from the Catholic Research Center, Melissa Shamini Perry, from the National University of Malaysia, Pauline Pooi Yin Leong and Yuen Beng Lee, both from Sunway University explore how the curtailing of physical religious activities during the pandemic impacted the psychological well-being of a group of Catholic older adults in Malaysia. There were concerns regarding how the sudden move to online religious activities would impact this group that is normally not technologically savvy and who rely on meaningful faith-based interactions in the community for their spiritual and psychological well-being. While common themes such as fear, anxiety, stress, feelings of isolation and anger were echoed, this group used positive religious coping strategies to deal with the initial setbacks in the practice of their faith. This helped them become more optimistic, flexible and empathetic towards others. The study discusses the link between positive religious coping strategies and better mental health outcomes when dealing with stressful life events.

In Chapter 6, *Factors promoting university instructor's resilience to technostress,* Chia Keat Yap from Asia Pacific University of Technology and Innovation and Si Na Kew from Universiti Technologi Malaysia process the impact of a heavily computer-mediated educational setting due to the transition of online learning in all educational institutions for a long period during the pandemic. They discuss a concept called 'technostress', which is measured by techno-load, techno-invasion, and techno-complexity on well-being. They also introduce how computer self-efficacy and positive self-esteem are resilience factors that mitigate against technostress. Improving contextual resilience factors and trait-like factors that enhance personal ability are practical measures recommended to buffer against technostress.

In Chapter 7, *The relationship between emotion regulation and well-being during the pandemic: Resilience as a mediator,* Nurul Izzah Fathiah binti Wan Ali Munawar and Eugene Y.J. Tee, both from HELP University, look at the mediating role of resilience in the relationship between emotion regulation strategies and well-being. Two emotion regulation strategies were explored, namely cognitive reappraisal and suppression. Resilience fully explained the relationship between reappraisal and well-being, but did not act as a mediator between suppression and well-being. In addition, while suppression as an emotion regulation strategy may provide some relief in the short term, unresolved emotions may have an impact on the well-being of a person in the longer term. Cognitive reappraisal, on the other hand, led to the development of resilience and an increased sense of well-being in a person. Cognitive reappraisal as an emotion regulation strategy was especially useful in periods of adversity and is recommended over the use of suppression during such times.

Acknowledgements

The editors of this book would like to acknowledge the fine work done by the authors of different chapters in this book. The insights into the psychological impact of COVID-19 in Malaysia will help policy makers and mental health practitioners to craft out strategies that will aid in the healing process of individuals and communities. Additional appreciation to a few authors, who also volunteered their time and effort as peer reviewers for other chapters in the book, namely Si Na Kew, Samuel Ern Hung Tsan, Azmawaty Mohamad Nor, Siew Li Ng, Hasse De Meyer, Pauline Pooi Yin Leong, Eugene Y.J. Tee and Chia Keat Yap. A special word of thanks also to peer reviewers from outside of this book project. They are academic scholars from the Department of Psychology at HELP University (Christopher Jit Meng Tan, Ai Hwa Quek, Timothy Tze Hao Liew, Elaine Fernandez, Karuna S. Thomas, TamilSelvan Ramis, Ho Yan Lai and Maria Felicitas Mamauag) and also from other institutions (Roy Rillera Marzo, Cynthia Shoba Anthony Thanaraj and Carlo Magno).

D. Gerard Joseph Louis
Surinderpal Kaur
Huey Fen Cheong

Section I

Working during the pandemic

1 Psychological distress among healthcare professionals at the frontlines

Anaesthesiologists' perspective

Samuel Ern Hung Tsan, Anand Kamalanathan, & Chew Yin Wang

1.1 Introduction

Amidst the COVID-19 pandemic, worldwide data indicated healthcare practitioners have a high incidence and prevalence of suffering from depression, burnout and anxiety, with multiple adverse consequences, such that it can be considered a "parallel pandemic" among healthcare workers. Burnout syndrome (BOS) is defined by the World Health Organization International Classification of Disease 11 (ICD 11) as a syndrome resulting from poorly managed chronic workplace stress (World Health Organization, 2019), while depression is defined as the presence of depressed mood or loss of interest in almost all activities in the ICD 11 (World Health Organization, 2020).

The prevalence of burnout and depression among healthcare practitioners in Malaysia has never been studied during a pandemic prior to this study. In the midst of the COVID-19 pandemic, this question has again been pushed into the forefront, due to concerns with maintaining the physical and mental wellbeing of clinicians handling this pandemic. At the same time, there is also no data on the factors associated with psychological distress among Malaysian medical workers, which is not desirable when planning for preventative strategies in alleviating their psychological distress. To answer these questions, we set forth to capture a snapshot of the situation in Malaysia with regards to burnout and depression among frontline anaesthesiology clinicians working in Sungai Buloh Hospital, the national infectious disease centre of Malaysia and the hospital gazetted to be an exclusive COVID-19 hospital in Malaysia.

With this study, more insight will be obtained into the psychological challenge that is faced by healthcare workers during pandemics by putting

DOI: 10.4324/9781003178576-2

the spotlight on the prevalence of burnout and depression. Also, by investigating the factors associated with burnout and depression, specific preventative strategies can be designed to improve the working conditions of Malaysian healthcare workers. Part of the data from our survey has been published as a correspondence article in the journal *Anaesthesia* (Tsan et al., 2020).

1.2 Literature review

The field of anaesthesiology and critical care has been specifically selected to be the target of the survey. This is due to the nature of work of anaesthesiologists in Malaysia, who handle the sickest patients in the intensive care unit (ICU) of the hospital. With regards to the pandemic, anaesthesiologists would be managing COVID-19 patients requiring airway management, life support equipment and medications, necessitating critical care in the ICU. Hence, they represent one of the groups of frontline healthcare practitioners most likely to suffer from burnout and depression.

1.2.1 Mental health in the field of anaesthesiology and critical care

The field of anaesthesiology and critical care is fraught with work-related psychological stress, where healthcare providers are faced with challenging ethical dilemmas, demanding daily responsibilities and high rate of patient mortality. In the midst of this work environment, the burnout syndrome (BOS) can occur (WHO, 2019). Multiple studies performed among anaesthesiologists and anaesthesia residents demonstrated that the prevalence of BOS working in such environments can be between 41% and 51% (de Oliveira et al., 2013; Sanfilippo et al., 2017; Sun et al., 2019). Similarly, critical care physicians are at increased risk of BOS, with studies showing a prevalence of 44% to 46.5% (Kerlin et al., 2020). This is a matter of great concern as BOS can cause posttraumatic stress disorder, alcohol abuse and even suicidal ideation (Dyrbye et al., 2008; Kerlin et al., 2020).

Research has shown that clinicians at all stages of their careers exhibit a higher level of depression than the general population. Prevalence of depression has been shown to be up to 60% in practicing clinicians (Bailey et al., 2018). In the field of anaesthesiology, trainees demonstrated high rates of depression, ranging from 12% to 18% (Looseley et al., 2019; Sun et al., 2019), while for anaesthesiologists up to 62.1% have been found to have depressive symptoms (Zhang, 2013). Similarly in the intensive care unit, physicians are at high risk of depression, with reported prevalence rate ranging from 18.8% to 23.8% (Embriaco et al., 2012; Garrouste-Orgeas et al., 2015). Aside from multiple adverse impacts on the emotional and physical health of clinicians, there could be implications for the safety of the practice of anaesthesiology and critical care, as depression has been found to be an independent risk factor for medical errors (Garrouste-Orgeas et al., 2015). In addition, anaesthesiology clinicians with higher burnout and depression risk are associated with less adherence to safety and practice standards (de Oliveira et al., 2013).

The phenomenon of burnout and depression among anaesthesiology clinicians is even more concerning in light of the current pandemic, which has led to increased workloads and stress for anaesthesiologists worldwide. In addition, the psychological pressure associated with increased risks of transmission of infections to clinicians may also contribute to risk of burnout and depression. A recent study on healthcare workers involving physicians and nurses who were exposed to COVID-19 patients in China showed that 50.4% of participants reported symptoms of depression, 44.6% had anxiety, 34.0% had insomnia and 71.5% reported distress (Lai et al., 2020). This is especially true for clinicians in the anaesthesiology field, who are currently serving on the front lines of the pandemic.

Prior to our survey being carried out, there was no data in the literature documenting the prevalence of burnout and depression among anaesthesiologists amidst the COVID-19 pandemic. This study was the first to bring to light this very important issue in Malaysia.

1.3 Methods

1.3.1 Participants

This study was approved by the Medical Research Ethics Committee of the Ministry of Health Malaysia. Throughout the whole month of May 2020, we conducted a cross-sectional survey of all clinicians ($n = 88$) in the Anaesthesiology and Intensive Care Department of Sungai Buloh Hospital (Tsan et al., 2020), which has been nationally gazetted as an exclusive COVID-19 hospital in Malaysia (Ram, 9 March 2020). All anaesthesiologists and anaesthesiology medical officers were eligible to participate, with the exception of those who refused to participate, or those who had been in the department for less than 1 month. All responses were anonymous and kept confidential. Written informed consent was obtained from subjects prior to participation in the survey. This study was prospectively registered on the Clinicaltrials.gov registry (Clinicaltrials.gov Identifier: NCT04362319).

1.3.2 Study measures

The study questionnaire consisted of 38 items, including demographics, social characteristics, working characteristics, burnout, symptoms of depression, self-perceived medical errors and worry of COVID-19 transmission. The survey was given by hand and collected in person after completion.

1.3.2.1 Burnout

Burnout was assessed with the physician-validated Maslach Burnout Inventory Human Services Survey (Medical Personnel) [MBI-HSS(MP)] (Maslach et al., 1996). The MBI-HSS (MP) contains 22 questions: 5 assessing depersonalisation, 9 for emotional exhaustion and 8 for personal accomplishment. A score was given to each question of the MBI-HSS (MP), based on a frequency scale of 0 "never" to 6 "every day". Similar to previous studies, participants with a high score in the sections on depersonalisation (DP) ($\geq$27) and/or emotional exhaustion (EE) ($\geq$10) were considered to have burnout (Dyrbye et al., 2009; Ma et al., 2019; Shanafelt et al., 2010; Tawfik et al., 2018; West et al., 2009).

1.3.2.2 Depression

The standardised 2-item Primary Care Evaluation of Mental Disorders (2-item PRIME-MD) questionnaire, which had been shown to perform as well as longer questionnaires, was used to evaluate for symptoms of depression (Spitzer et al., 1994; Whooley et al., 1997). The 2-item PRIME-MD questionnaire was selected as it had been found to be a useful screening test for depression with high sensitivity, and is less time consuming. Any "Yes" answer to either of the following two questions would be considered a positive test: (1) "During the past month, have you often been bothered by feeling down, depressed, or hopeless?" or (2) "During the past month, have you often been bothered by little interest or pleasure in doing things?"

1.3.2.3 Self-perceived medical errors

In order to evaluate self-perceived medical errors that occurred over the past 1 month, similar to previous studies, two questions were asked with the purpose of finding out recent events that have been internalised as a major medical error by the clinician (Shanafelt et al., 2010; Tawfik et al., 2018; West et al., 2006). The first question in this section was "Are you concerned you have made any major medical errors in the last one month?" For those who answered "yes" to this question, the follow-up question was "Which of the following was the single greatest contributing factor in this particular error?" The response options for this follow-up question will be: (a) system issue (e.g., someone misinterpreted an order); (b) your degree of fatigue; (c) lapse in your concentration; (d) lapse in judgment; (e) lack of knowledge; (f) your degree of stress/burnout; (g) other (free text).

1.3.2.4 *Worry of COVID-19 transmission*

Worry of COVID-19 transmission was asked as a single question, with responses graded using a numerical rating scale (NRS), "0" being not worried at all while a score of "10" signifies worst worry possible. The NRS has been validated to assess anxiety, and hence we adapted it to assess for worry of COVID-19 (Walawender et al., 2015). Cronbach alpha value for the questionnaire combining all these items was 0.791, indicating good internal consistency.

1.3.3 *Statistical analysis*

A minimum sample size of 78 clinicians in the Anaesthesiology and Intensive Care Department was required to have a confidence level of 99%, with a 5% margin of error, in order that the results obtained would accurately reflect the population of interest. Standard descriptive statistics were performed to summarise the demographic and baseline characteristic variables. Associations between variables were investigated using Pearson chi-square test, the independent samples t-test or the Mann-Whitney U test as appropriate. The normality of distribution for continuous variables was determined via the Shapiro-Wilk test. Multivariate logistic regression was conducted to determine factors that were independently associated with burnout and depression risk, by utilising the "Enter" selection method. The variables included in the model for burnout included number of calls per week, worry about COVID-19 and depression risk, while the model for depression risk included the same variables plus age factor. All tests were two-sided, and type 1 error probability alpha value was set at 0.05. All statistical analyses were performed with SPSS version 22.0 (SPSS Inc. Chicago, IL, USA).

1.4 Findings

A total of 88 questionnaires were distributed to all anaesthesiology clinicians in the Department of Anaesthesiology and Critical Care of Sungai Buloh Hospital, of which 85 (96.6%) were completed and returned (Tsan et al., 2020). The three anaesthesiologists who were not included declined to participate in the survey. Respondent characteristics are summarised in Table 1.1.

Table 1.1 Respondents' (anaesthesiologists') characteristics (*n* = 85)

Age (in years)[a]	31 (28–36)
Gender[a]	
Male	31 (36.5)
Female	54 (63.5)
Anaesthetic experience (in years)[a]	3 (1 – 8)
Anaesthesia training level[a]	
Medical officer	62 (72.9)
Consultant	23 (27.1)
Hours of work per week (in hours)[a]	
< 50	41 (48.2)
50–59	22 (25.9)
60–69	22 (25.9)
No of calls per week[a]	
0–1	26 (30.6)
≥ 2	59 (69.4)
Frequency of handling Covid-19 patients[a]	
Daily	80 (94.1)
Weekly or monthly	5 (5.9)
Marital status	
Yes	46 (54.1)
No	39 (45.9)
Parental status	
Yes	41 (48.2)
No	44 (51.8)
Alcohol status	
Yes	13 (15.3)
No	72 (84.7)
Smoking status	
Yes	3 (3.5)
No	82 (96.5)

Abbreviations: IQR, Interquartile range; *n*, number.

[a] Data previously published (Tsan et al., 2020).

1.4.1 Baseline characteristics

The median age of respondents was 31 years, and the majority were women (63.5%). Medical officers make up the majority of anaesthesiology clinicians who participated, with respondents having a median 3 years of anaesthetic work experience. During this pandemic, approximately 52% participants were working more than 50 hours per week, with the majority (69.4%) doing at least two calls per week. Up to 94.1% of those who participated handled COVID-19 patients daily (Tsan et al., 2020).

1.4.2 Outcome measures

Characteristics of respondents with respect to burnout, depression risk, worry of COVID-19 and self-perceived medical errors are summarised in Table 1.2.

Table 1.2 Burnout, depression risk, worry about COVID-19 and medical errors among respondents (*n* = 85)

Burnout indices[e]	
Emotional exhaustion[a]	
Mean (SD)	21.35 (9.9)
Low	29 (34.1)
Intermediate	29 (34.1)
High	27 (31.8)
Depersonalisation[b]	
Mean (SD)	8.74 (4.9)
Low	18 (21.2)
Intermediate	27 (31.8)
High	40 (47.1)
Personal accomplishment[c]	
Mean (SD)	29.2 (7.4)
Low	54 (63.5)
Intermediate	23 (27.1)
High	8 (9.4)
Burnout[e]	
Yes	47 (55.3)
No	38 (44.7)
Depression risk[e]	
Yes	57 (67.1)
No	28 (32.9)
Worry about Covid-19[d,e]	
Median (IQR)	7 (5–8)
Mild	11 ((12.9)
Moderate	40 (47.1)
Major	34 (40.0)
Medical errors	
Yes	37 (43.5)
No	48 (56.5)
Greatest contributing factor in medical error	
System issue	1 (2.2)
Fatigue	3 (6.7)
Lapse in concentration	10 (22.2)
Lapse in judgment	13 (28.9)
Lack of knowledge	14 (31.1)
Stress/burnout	3 (6.7)
PPE-related	1 (2.2)

(*Continued*)

Table 1.2 Burnout, depression risk, worry about COVID-19 and
medical errors among respondents (*n* = 85)   (*Continued*)

Results in *n* (%) unless stated otherwise.

Abbreviations: IQR, interquartile range; *n*, number; PPE, personal protective
equipment; SD, standard deviation.

[a] Emotional exhaustion scoring: low < 18, intermediate 18–26, high ≥ 27.
Higher score denotes higher degree of burnout.

[b] Depersonalisation scoring: low ≤ 4, intermediate 5–9, high ≥ 10. Higher
score denotes higher degree of burnout.

[c] Personal accomplishment scoring: low ≤ 32, intermediate 33–39, high ≥ 40.
Lower score denotes higher degree of burnout.

[d] Worry about Covid-19 stratified based on: Mild (scores 0–4), Moderate
(scores 5–7), Major (scores 8–10).

[e] Data previously published (Tsan et al., 2020).

A total of 31.8% had high emotional exhaustion, 47.1% had high depersonalisation and 63.5% had low personal accomplishment. Overall, 55.3% were classified as burnout based on high scores in the emotional exhaustion and/or depersonalisation indices. Among all the respondents, 67.1% demonstrated depression risk. Up to 40% reported having major worry about COVID-19 amidst the pandemic (Tsan et al., 2020). The rates of self-perceived medical errors in the past 1 month during the COVID-19 situation was up to 43.5%, with the greatest contributing factors being lapse in judgment, lack of knowledge and lapse in concentration. Of note, one respondent reported committing a medical error due to the use of personal protective equipment.

1.4.3 Factors associated with burnout and depression

No demographic and social factors were significantly associated with burnout and depression risk. Burnout and depression risk were significantly associated with each other ($\chi^2 = 15.502$, $p < 0.001$) (Figure 1.1) (Tsan et al., 2020). Both burnout and depression risk were also associated with the number of calls per week ($\chi^2 = 4.293$, $p = 0.038$ and $\chi^2 = 4.935$, $p = 0.026$, respectively) (Figure 1.1) (Tsan et al., 2020).

In assessing the association of burnout and depression risk with worry of COVID-19, the Mann-Whitney test was utilised as the results indicated a non-normal distribution. Burnout and depression risk were significantly associated with worry of COVID-19 (Mann-Whitney U = 620, $p = 0.014$ and Mann-Whitney U = 586, $p = 0.044$, respectively) (Figure 1.2) (Tsan et al., 2020).

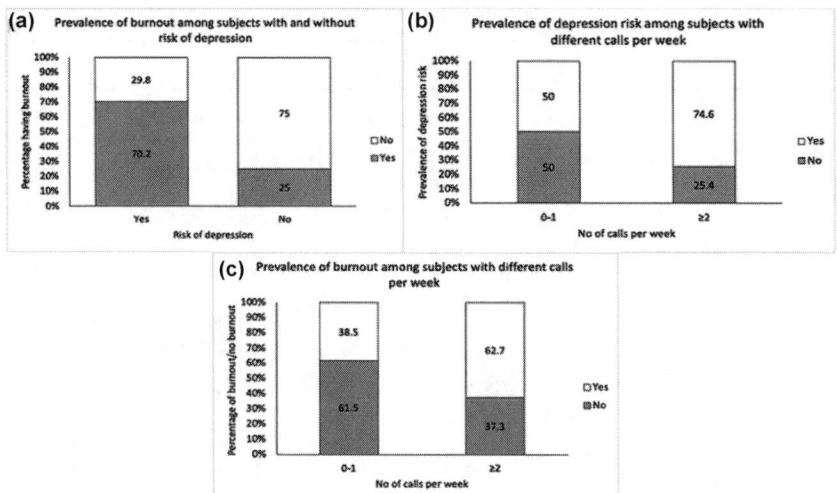

Figure 1.1 Factors associated with anaesthesiologists' burnout and depression risk: (a) burnout vs. depression risk ($p < 0.0001$); (b) number of calls vs. depression risk ($p = 0.026$) and (c) number of calls vs. burnout ($p = 0.038$).

Rates of self-perceived medical error was not significantly associated with both burnout and depression risk. In multivariate analysis, only burnout and depression were independently associated with each other, with respondents who are burnout more likely to be depressed and vice versa (Table 1.3).

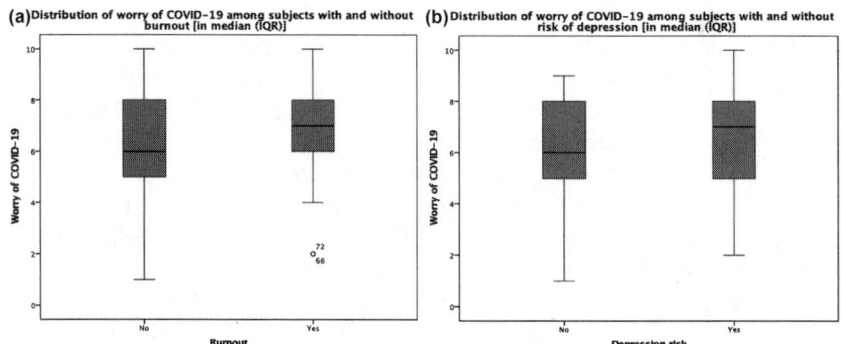

Figure 1.2 Association between anaesthesiologists' worry of COVID-19 with (a) burnout ($p = 0.014$) and (b) depression risk ($p = 0.044$).

Table 1.3 Multivariate logistic regression analysis for burnout and depression risk

Burnout				
Factors	*Crude OR[a] (95% CI)*	*p value*	*Adjusted OR[a] (95% CI)*	*p value*
No of calls per week[b]	2.69 (1.04–6.96)	0.041	1.82 (0.62–5.33)	0.274
Worry of Covid-19[c]	1.32 (1.06–1.64)	0.015	1.24 (0.97–1.58)	0.090
Depression risk[d]	7.06 (2.53–19.70)	< 0.001	5.63 (1.95–16.30)	0.001
Depression risk				
Factors	*Crude OR[a] (95% CI)*	*p value*	*Adjusted OR[a] (95% CI)*	*p value*
Age[c]	0.91 (0.83–0.997)	0.043	0.89 (0.79–1.00)	0.049
No of calls per week[b]	2.93 (1.12–7.71)	0.029	1.97 (0.66–5.90)	0.227
Worry of Covid-19[c]	1.27 (1.01–1.58)	0.037	1.26 (0.95–1.68)	0.110
Burnout[e]	7.06 (2.53–19.70)	< 0.001	4.95 (1.65–14.80)	0.004

Abbreviations: CI, confidence interval; No, number; OR, odds ratio.

[a] OR > 1 indicates higher risk of burnout/depression risk, OR < 1 indicates lower risk of burnout/depression risk.
[b] ≥ 2 calls per week compared to 0–1 call per week.
[c] Measured on continuous scale.
[d] Depression risk compared to no depression risk.
[e] Burnout compared to no burnout.

1.5 Conclusion

Our study is among the first to look at burnout and depression risk in the anaesthesiology fraternity during a worldwide pandemic. Our findings, though not unexpected, showed that a "parallel pandemic" of emotional harm to anaesthesiologists is not just a theoretical postulation, but is indeed the case during the COVID-19 pandemic (Dzau et al., 13 May 2020). We found that more than half of anaesthesiology clinicians in our survey have burnout and depression risk, with clinicians who experience burnout more likely to be depressed and vice versa. In addition, burnout and depression risk are associated with the number of calls per week, and also worry of COVID-19. Up to 40% of anaesthesiologists reported having major worry of being infected by COVID-19. The rates of medical errors during this pandemic is also worryingly high, with up to 43.5% reporting experiencing medical errors in this time of crisis. Our findings have been subsequently confirmed in a similar Italian study by Magnavita et al. (2020) where up to 71.1% of anaesthesiologists reported high work-related stress, 36.7% reported having insomnia, 27.8% had anxiety and 51.1% had depression.

1.5.1 *Potential causes of high prevalence of burnout and depression*

In view of the central role the anaesthesiology field is playing during this worldwide pandemic, the high prevalence of burnout and depression risk is not surprising (Magnavita et al., 2020; Sasangohar et al., 2020). Although surgical caseload in the operating theatre decreased, anaesthesiology clinicians' workload have not reduced, but may have instead increased as the number of COVID-19 patients increased. This is demonstrated in our survey when we found almost 70% of respondents had at least 2 calls per week, and almost 52% worked at least 50 hours per week. This compares well with the study by Magnavita et al. (2020), which found that 63% of anaesthesiologists reported increased or much increased workloads.

The role of the anaesthesiologists in the pandemic is to manage patients in acute and critical care, with special emphasis on airway management, ventilation support, oxygen therapy, hemodynamic management, analgesia and sedation (Zhang et al., 2020). As the clinician responsible for airway management, anaesthesiologists are among those at greatest risk of contracting COVID-19, due to the aerosolisation nature of intubation (Meng et al., 2020). In our centre during this pandemic, as is the case with many other hospitals in Malaysia, anaesthesiology clinicians form intubation teams for critically ill COVID-19 patients, attending to multiple patients in a day. Although the situation in Malaysia is not as dire as in China or in other more heavily affected countries, anaesthesiologists in Malaysia are central in the teams that have been called "coronavirus intubation team racing against death" (Huaxia, 2020; Zhang et al., 2020).

With this frequent exposure to COVID-19, the respondents in our survey reported a median score of 7 for worry about COVID-19 on a numerical rating scale of 10, and up to 40% reported major worry of this virus. This is a potential cause of the high prevalence of burnout and depression seen in this population. Also, the mental burden of facing increased patient morbidity and mortality due to COVID-19 in critically ill patients is substantial, and would also contribute to burnout and depression risk (Kerlin et al., 2020; Moss et al., 2016). Our survey demonstrated a snapshot of the unique and dire circumstances anaesthesiologists in Malaysia find themselves in amidst the COVID-19 pandemic, and to a certain extent by other healthcare practitioners at the frontlines of the battle against the virus.

1.5.2 *Impact on medical errors*

At the turn of the century, there has been an exponential increase in awareness of the impact of medical error and patient safety. In our survey, approximately 44% of anaesthesiology clinicians reported experiencing medical errors in the preceding 1 month during the pandemic. Medical error is a global problem that results in patient harm and increased healthcare costs (Kohn et al., 1999). This problem is compounded by the pandemic, with its unique challenges in terms of increased workload, severely ill patient condition and fear of cross infection, to name a few. The high prevalence of self-perceived medical errors we found amidst this pandemic should serve as a trigger for further research into the rates of medical errors, the causes and the potential recommendations to improve patient safety.

Although we did not find a relationship between burnout and depression with medical errors likely due to insufficient power of the study, many studies have shown that they are linked to each other (Moss et al., 2016; Shanafelt et al., 2010; Tawfik et al., 2018). A meta-analysis of 42,473 physicians found that burnout was associated with a 2-fold increase in odds for patient safety incidents and poorer quality of care due to low professionalism (Panagioti et al., 2018). The relationship between burnout and medical errors may be a bidirectional one, with errors leading to stress and subsequently burnout, while burnout may lead to reduced performance and thus more errors (Kerlin et al., 2020; Moss et al., 2016). This potential vicious cycle is even more concerning in light of the current pandemic, and serves as a wake-up call to all healthcare professionals.

1.5.3 Interventions

Amidst this "parallel pandemic" of emotional stress in the form of burnout and depression, emphasis should be placed on solutions and improvements. Interventions can be classified into four main categories; physician level, organisation level, national level and international level (Dzau et al., 13 May 2020).

As a first step, efforts should be made to educate the medical fraternity on burnout and depression via campaigns, continuing medical education sessions and the mass media. Recognition of the problem is crucial in managing this "parallel pandemic". As more and more medical workers recognise the high prevalence of burnout and depression, and understand the impacts on their work and personal life, they will be more willing to seek help.

On the organisation level, Shanafelt et al. (2020) reported that physicians' requests to organisations were to hear, protect, prepare, support and care for physicians amidst the pandemic (Shanafelt et al., 2020). Organisational leaders and employers should take steps to do regular monthly or bimonthly assessments to detect burnout and depression amongst their staff. A chief wellness officer in the highest executive level should be appointed and tasked with the detection and management of those with burnout and depression, in addition to carrying out programs to prevent these psychological adverse effects from developing (Tsan et al., 2020). Those with ability to make decisions should actively encourage a good work–life balance. Furthermore, peer support groups should be set up, to allow those with prior experience of burnout and depression to help their colleagues.

On the national level, the government has a role in ensuring mental health programs are appropriately funded amidst the pandemic. Additional financial remunerations can also be provided to those serving at the frontlines who are putting their lives at risk in managing COVID-19 patients.

On the international stage, world health bodies need to place more emphasis on the mental wellbeing of medical workers, and find ways to collaborate more closely with each other with regards to sharing information and practices to alleviate psychological distress among healthcare workers (Tsan et al., 2020)

1.5.4 Limitations of the study

Our study had a few limitations. Firstly, this survey was conducted in a single centre, an exclusively COVID-19 patients hospital, and hence the results may not be generalisable. We decided not to include other hybrid hospitals managing COVID-19 and non COVID-19 patients, in order to reduce the number of confounders. In this study, we sought to demonstrate one end of the extreme, namely the prevalence of burnout and depression among anaesthesiology clinicians who are solely managing COVID-19 patients. Secondly, this was a cross-sectional study, and therefore we were unable to show any causality in the relationships. Similarly due to the nature of cross-sectional studies, we acknowledge that burnout and depression are affected by numerous factors, many of which may not have been measured in the study. Thirdly, our study is likely underpowered to detect many of the associations between various factors with burnout and depression. Nevertheless, this is among the first studies looking at the mental and emotional burdens shouldered by anaesthesiologists during a pandemic, and is a stepping stone to further large-scale research into this underrecognised yet critical issue.

The snapshot of the high prevalence of burnout and depression risk among clinicians in the Anaesthesiology Department does raise questions about what might be happening to other healthcare professionals working in the frontlines of the pandemic. Further research should be carried out to determine if this scenario is prevalent in the whole of Malaysia, and to identify factors contributing to this phenomenon. Efforts should be made in Malaysia's health system to address these serious issues and find appropriate solutions before further harm ensues.

Practical suggestions

Burnout and depression among healthcare practitioners in Malaysia amidst the COVID-19 pandemic is a pressing issue with wide-ranging repercussions, and hence a concerted effort is required to recognise and address this important problem. Empowering medical professionals' mental resilience and fortitude is crucial in turning the tide against the COVID-19 virus.

References

Bailey, E., Robinson, J., & McGorry, P. (2018). Depression and suicide among medical practitioners in Australia. *Internal Medicine Journal, 48*(3), 254–258.

de Oliveira, G. S. Jr, Chang, R., Fitzgerald, P. C., Almeida, M. D., Castro-Alves, L. S., Ahmad, S., & McCarthy, R. J. (2013). The prevalence of burnout and depression and their association with adherence to safety and practice standards: A survey of United States anesthesiology trainees. *Anesthesia & Analgesia, 117*(1), 182–193.

Dyrbye, L. N., Thomas, M. R., Massie, F. S., Power, D. V., Eacker, A., Harper, W., Durning, S., Moutier, C., Szydlo, D. W., & Novotny, P. J. (2008). Burnout and suicidal ideation among US medical students. *Annals of Internal Medicine, 149*(5), 334–341.

Dyrbye, L. N., West, C. P., & Shanafelt, T. D. (2009). Defining burnout as a dichotomous variable. *Journal of General Internal Medicine, 24*(3), 440.

Dzau, V. J., Kirch, D., & Nasca, T. (13 May 2020). Preventing a parallel pandemic – a national strategy to protect clinicians' well-being. *New England Journal of Medicine.* Retrieved 20 June 2020 from https://www.nejm.org/doi/full/10.1056/nejmp2011027

Embriaco, N., Hraiech, S., Azoulay, E., Baumstarck-Barrau, K., Forel, J.-M., Kentish-Barnes, N., Pochard, F., Loundou, A., Roch, A., & Papazian, L. (2012). Symptoms of depression in ICU physicians. *Annals of Intensive Care, 2*(1), 34.

Garrouste-Orgeas, M., Perrin, M., Soufir, L., Vesin, A., Blot, F., Maxime, V., Beuret, P., Troché, G., Klouche, K., & Argaud, L. (2015). The iatroref study: Medical errors are associated with symptoms of depression in ICU staff but not burnout or safety culture. *Intensive Care Medicine, 41*(2), 273–284.

Huaxia. (2020, 25 February 2020). Coronavirus fight: A race against death! Intubation team in Wuhan do utmost to save patients. *Xinhuanet News.* Retrieved 20 June 2020 from http://www.xinhuanet.com/english/2020-02/25/c_138817011.htm, https://www.youtube.com/watch?v=544pGYpAKUA

Kerlin, M. P., McPeake, J., & Mikkelsen, M. E. (2020). Burnout and joy in the profession of critical care medicine. *Critical Care, 24*, 1–6.

Kohn, L. T., Corrigan, J., & Donaldson, M. S. (1999). *To err is human: Building a safer health system.* National Academy Press.

Lai, J., Ma, S., Wang, Y., Cai, Z., Hu, J., Wei, N., Wu, J., Du, H., Chen, T., & Li, R. (2020). Factors associated with mental health outcomes among health care workers exposed to coronavirus disease 2019. *JAMA Network Open*, *3*(3), e203976–e203976.

Looseley, A., Wainwright, E., Cook, T. M., Bell, V., Hoskins, S., O'Connor, M., Taylor, G., & Mouton, R. (2019). Stress, burnout, depression and work-satisfaction amongst UK anaesthetic trainees: A quantitative analysis of the satisfaction and wellbeing in anaesthetic trainee study. *Anaesthesia*, *74*(10), 1231–1239.

Ma, S., Huang, Y., Yang, Y., Ma, Y., Zhou, T., Zhao, H., Chen, L., Zhou, N., & Zhang, L. (2019). Prevalence of burnout and career satisfaction among oncologists in China: A national survey. *The Oncologist*, *24*(7), e480–e489.

Magnavita, N., Soave, P. M., Ricciardi, W., & Antonelli, M. (2020). Occupational stress and mental health among anesthetists during the COVID-19 pandemic. *International Journal of Environmental Research and Public Health*, *17*, 8245.

Maslach, C., Jackson, S. E., & Leiter, M. P. (1996). *Maslach burnout inventory* (3rd ed., Vol. 21). Palo Alto, CA: Consulting Psychologists.

Meng, L., Qiu, H., Wan, L., Ai, Y., Xue, Z., Guo, Q., Deshpande, R., Zhang, L., Meng, J., & Tong, C. (2020). Intubation and ventilation amid the COVID-19 outbreak: Wuhan's experience. *Anesthesiology*, *132*(6), 1317–1332.

Moss, M., Good, V. S., Gozal, D., Kleinpell, R., & Sessler, C. N. (2016). A critical care societies collaborative statement: Burnout syndrome in critical care healthcare professionals. A call for action. *American Journal of Respiratory and Critical Care Medicine*, *194*(1), 106–113.

Panagioti, M., Geraghty, K., Johnson, J., Zhou, A., Panagopoulou, E., Chew-Graham, C., Peters, D., Hodkinson, A., Riley, R., & Esmail, A. (2018). Association between physician burnout and patient safety, professionalism, and patient satisfaction: A systematic review and meta-analysis. *JAMA Internal Medicine*, *178*(10), 1317–1331.

Ram, B. S. (9 March 2020). *Health Ministry ready to face surge in COVID-19 cases*. Retrieved 19 April 2020 from https://www.nst.com.my/news/nation/2020/03/573205/health-ministry-ready-face-surge-COVID-19-cases

Sanfilippo, F., Noto, A., Foresta, G., Santonocito, C., Palumbo, G. J., Arcadipane, A., Maybauer, D. M., & Maybauer, M. O. (2017). Incidence and factors associated with burnout in anesthesiology: A systematic review. *BioMed Research International*, Volume 2017, Article ID 8648925, 10 pages.

Sasangohar, F., Jones, S. L., Masud, F. N., Vahidy, F. S., & Kash, B. A. (2020). Provider burnout and fatigue during the COVID-19 pandemic: Lessons learned from a high-volume intensive care unit. *Anesthesia and Analgesia*, *131*(1), 106–111.

Shanafelt, T. D., Balch, C. M., Bechamps, G., Russell, T., Dyrbye, L., Satele, D., Collicott, P., Novotny, P. J., Sloan, J., & Freischlag, J. (2010). Burnout and medical errors among American surgeons. *Annals of Surgery*, *251*(6), 995–1000.

Shanafelt, T., Ripp, J., & Trockel, M. (2020). Understanding and addressing sources of anxiety among health care professionals during the COVID-19 pandemic. *JAMA*, *323*(21), 2133–2134.

Spitzer, R. L., Williams, J. B. W., Kroenke, K., Linzer, M., deGruy, F. V., Hahn, S. R., Brody, D., & Johnson, J. G. (1994). Utility of a new procedure for diagnosing mental disorders in primary care: The PRIME-MD 1000 study. *JAMA*, *272*(22), 1749–1756.

Sun, H., Warner, D. O., Macario, A., Zhou, Y., Culley, D. J., & Keegan, M. T. (2019). Repeated cross-sectional surveys of burnout, distress, and depression among anesthesiology residents and first-year graduates. *Anesthesiology*, *131*(3), 668–677.

Tawfik, D. S., Profit, J., Morgenthaler, T. I., Satele, D. V., Sinsky, C. A., Dyrbye, L. N., Tutty, M. A., West, C. P., & Shanafelt, T. D. (2018). Physician burnout, well-being, and work unit safety grades in relationship to reported medical errors. *Mayo Clinic Proceedings*, *93*(11), 1571–1580.

Tsan, S. E. H., Kamalanathan, A., Lee, C. K., Zakaria, S. A., & Wang, C. Y. (2020). A survey on burnout and depression risk among anaesthetists during COVID-19: The tip of an iceberg? *Anaesthesia*, *76*(Suppl 3), 8–10.

Walawender, I., Roczniak, W., Nowak, D., Skowron, M., Waliczek, M., Rogalska, A., & Nowak, P. G. (2015). Applicability of the numeric scale for anxiety evaluation in patients undergoing dental treatment. *Dental and Medical Problems*, *52*(2), 205–214.

West, C. P., Dyrbye, L. N., Sloan, J. A., & Shanafelt, T. D. (2009). Single item measures of emotional exhaustion and depersonalization are useful for assessing burnout in medical professionals. *Journal of General Internal Medicine*, *24*(12), 1318–1321.

West, C. P., Huschka, M. M., Novotny, P. J., Sloan, J. A., Kolars, J. C., Habermann, T. M., & Shanafelt, T. D. (2006). Association of perceived medical errors with resident distress and empathy: A prospective longitudinal study. *JAMA*, *296*(9), 1071–1078.

Whooley, M. A., Avins, A. L., Miranda, J., & Browner, W. S. (1997). Case-finding instruments for depression: Two questions are as good as many. *Journal of General Internal Medicine*, *12*(7), 439–445.

World Health Organization. (2019). *Burn-out*. Retrieved 10 June 2020 from https://icd.who.int/browse11/l-m/en#/http://id.who.int/icd/entity/129180281

World Health Organization. (2020). *Single episode depressive disorder*. Retrieved 10 June 2020 from https://icd.who.int/browse11/l-m/en#/http://id.who.int/icd/entity/578635574

Zhang, H.-F., Bo, L., Lin, Y., Li, F.-X., Sun, S., Lin, H.-B., Xu, S.-Y., Bian, J., Yao, S., & Chen, X. (2020). Response of Chinese anesthesiologists to the COVID-19 outbreak. *Anesthesiology*, *132*(6), 1333–1338.

Zhang, Y. (2013). Work condition, work-related stress, fatigue and depressive symptoms among Chinese anesthetists. *British Journal of Anaesthesia*, *111*, eLetters Supplement.

2 Psychological distress among essential and non-essential service workers

Marc Archer & Chee Hoong Moey

2.1 Introduction

With the spread of the global pandemic during early-to-mid 2020 came a widespread shift away from the workplace to reduce exposure and contagion (Shah et al., 2020). However, this 'new normal' of remote meetings and home offices was not universal, and a large proportion of the workforce was required to continue going to work with elevated risks (The Lancet, 2020). Healthcare providers and other essential service workers who were required to be in contact with the public have shown elevated levels of psychological distress, such as symptoms of anxiety and depression (Giorgi et al., 2020).

The study reported in this chapter was developed to determine the prevalence of psychological distress across the Malaysian workforce, and compare those employed in essential and non-essential services as defined by the Malaysian government to cover the first period of the Movement Control Order (MCO)[1] starting March 18, 2020. The secondary objective was to identify associations with any specific pandemic-related behaviours (e.g. taking precautions) and concerns (e.g. becoming infected). Findings from the current research can inform targeted public mental health messaging, human resource management, and a range of psychological interventions.

2.2 Literature review

2.2.1 Psychological distress during the COVID-19 pandemic

A nationally representative survey of the general adult population conducted in China during the peak of the local epidemic identified sharp rises in anxiety and depression (increasing from approximately 4% in pre-pandemic 2019 to around 20% in February 2020; Li et al., 2020).

DOI: 10.4324/9781003178576-3

Studies in other countries, also undertaken during initial phases of lockdown, found similarly elevated figures (e.g. Hyland et al., 2020 for the Republic of Ireland).

However, observed increases were less drastic in countries with typically higher pre-pandemic rates of anxiety/depression, for example in the UK (Shevlin et al., 2020), and Spain (Valiente et al., 2021). While pre-pandemic data on prevalence of anxiety and depression among Malaysians is limited, it has been estimated at relatively moderate levels of around 8% and 12%, respectively (e.g. Sherina et al., 2012) and so we might expect similarly moderate increases resulting from the pandemic.

Across studies, concerns specific to COVID-19 have predicted higher levels of general anxiety and depression (e.g. Li et al., 2020; Valiente et al., 2021). Higher perceived risk of infection is also commonly found to be associated with higher levels of anxiety and depression. Thus, those working in roles with greater exposure to individuals who are infected or of unknown infection status may be at particularly high risk of psychological distress. Given the often lifesaving necessity of medical provision during the pandemic, by comparison to non-healthcare essential service workers (such as those in transportation and food supply), essential service workers in healthcare roles have received pronounced media and research attention (e.g. Mehta et al., 2021). Accordingly, it is important to delineate how COVID-19 might have differentially affected those in both healthcare and non-healthcare essential services.

2.2.2 *Impact on essential service workers*

2.2.2.1 *Healthcare essential service workers*

While early data from China indicated an association between proximity to infected individuals and mental health risk among healthcare workers (Lai et al., 2020), such data were lacking for the Malaysian context. Recently published work, however, indicates a large burden on Malaysian healthcare workers with over half experiencing burnout between April and May 2020 (Roslan et al., 2021).

A five-nation study also including India, Indonesia, Singapore and Vietnam found levels of depression (14.3%) and anxiety (14.9%) among healthcare workers in Malaysia during the pandemic to be significantly higher than in these other countries (none higher than 6.7% and 6.8%, respectively) between April and June 2020 (Chew et al., 2020). The reason for such elevated levels of psychological distress is not clear, particularly in relation to neighbouring and highly similar Singapore which also had high levels of testing and low COVID-19 case numbers, and requires closer investigation.

However, it is also unclear if elevated psychological distress is associated with an essential service role or the general background concerns of the pandemic. Indeed, a systematic review across 5 studies (4 from China, 1 from Singapore) involving 6,035 healthcare workers and 5,417 non-healthcare workers found no significant difference between groups in levels of anxiety and depression (Sheraton et al., 2020).

The single Singapore-based study included in Sheraton et al.'s (2020) review, which might provide greatest comparability to Malaysia, tested differences between medical and non-medical healthcare workers providing a more nuanced insight as the former are expected to have highest proximity to infected patients (Tan et al., 2020). Perhaps counter-intuitively the data found medical healthcare workers to have significantly lower levels of anxiety than non-medical healthcare workers (10.8% vs 20.7%). The authors suggest that this might be due to levels of mental preparedness, understanding of medical risk and training around PPE use and infection control. In short, expertise and role may serve as protective factors despite proximity to the disease.

2.2.2.2 *Non-healthcare essential service workers*

As noted above, much less is known about the risk of psychological distress among non-healthcare essential service workers. This dearth of research is conspicuous and concerning, particularly as a nationwide survey in Australia conducted in April 2020 found that, while healthcare essential workers actually had lower levels of anxiety and depression than those in the general population, those working in non-healthcare essential services reported the highest levels of all (Toh et al., 2021). In light of Tan et al.'s (2020) finding that medical healthcare workers might be at reduced risk due to possible exposure being countered by insight, training and mental preparedness, the exceptional susceptibility to elevated psychological distress among those in essential services entirely outside of healthcare professions might arise from the combined increased exposure and minimal protective resources.

2.2.3 *Impact on non-essential service workers*

While the MCO should mean that those working in non-essential services have relatively reduced exposure to contagion, and thus reduced risk of related psychological distress, a different set of constraints (e.g. reduced work/life boundaries, virtual communication) and concerns (e.g. job insecurity, general pandemic threat) have emerged (see Kniffin et al. 2021, for a review). In addition to the non-zero risk of infection, and related concerns for friends and family, many in non-essential services have experienced increased childcare duties and unplanned shifts in job demands (e.g. Xiao et al., 2021). Although previous research has not focused on the workforce specifically, a general survey of Malaysians during the first phase of the MCO indicated that threat to personal/family health and economic impact of an indefinitely prolonged crisis were greatest sources of stress (Mahmud et al., 2020).

Accordingly, the current study sought to better understand how specific behaviours and concerns around working amidst the pandemic might be associated with psychological distress among the Malaysian workforce with a specific focus on non-healthcare essential service workers.

2.3 Method

2.3.1 Research approach

The study employed a cross-sectional self-report online survey to provide an indication of contemporaneous psychological distress across the Malaysian workforce.

2.3.2 Participants

The participants were recruited to the study via social media posts, emails and word of mouth within organisations supporting the study. The only inclusion criterion was being aged at least 18 years, and there were no exclusion criteria. A priori power analysis using G*Power (with alpha level: 0.05 and power: 0.80) indicated a minimal sample size of 164 to detect medium effect sizes of 0.3.

2.3.3 Procedure

Ethics approval was obtained from HELP University's Department of Psychology Ethics Review Board prior to commencement of the study. The study was advertised widely through existing workplace communication channels at approximately 30 organisations of diverse size (tens to thousands of employees) and type (including universities, supermarkets, and delivery services) between mid-May to mid-August 2020. Request to participate in surveys is normal within the workplace, and it was made clear that this study aims to better understand the experiences and needs of employees across Malaysia during the COVID-19 pandemic and the

MCO. Separate advertisements were circulated in English and Bahasa Malaysia, with links leading into study materials in that same language. Those who clicked on the link were provided with detailed information on the study, invited to ask questions, and required to provide consent to take part.

2.3.4 Measures

Working within an essential service was determined by responses to two items in a sociodemographic questionnaire. The first binary item asked, 'Are you employed within an essential service, e.g. food supply, healthcare, transport?' with a list of such services as provided by the Malaysian government (as cited above, and see endnote) from which participants responding 'yes' had to select. All demographic items were developed in English and then translated into Bahasa Malaysia through standard back-translation.

Depression and anxiety symptoms were measured using the Patient Health Questionnaire (PHQ-9; Kroenke et al., 2001) and Generalized Anxiety Disorder (GAD-7; Spitzer et al., 2006) scale respectively. These two widely used and well-validated measures were selected for comparability to other surveys of psychological distress. As the survey was made available in both English and Bahasa Malaysia, validated Bahasa Malaysia versions of the PHQ-9 (Sherina et al., 2012) and GAD-7 were used (Sidik et al., 2012). Cronbach's alphas for the current study were 0.90 and 0.93, respectively, indicating excellent internal consistency.

Pandemic-related concerns were measured with a 16-item self-report questionnaire created specifically for the current study and called, for convenience, the Behaviours and Concerns Amidst Pandemic Scale (BCAPS). A review of the literature determined that there was no standardised and validated measure of perceived risk of contagion and pandemic-related concerns. Given the urgency to gather data amidst the pandemic, which does not allow for formal scale development and validation, this approach uses each item on the BCAPS as a discrete variable. Generated through consultation with experts working in the healthcare system, the first five items begin with the stem 'During this period, for work purposes I...' and include 'am at risk of being infected' and 'take precautions to reduce risk of infection'. Indications of frequency are given on a 5-point Likert scale ranging from 0 = *never* to 4 = *almost always*. The remaining 11 items all start with the stem 'During this period, I have been concerned about' with areas of concern including 'becoming infected myself' *and* 'others perceiving me as "contagious"'. All items were developed in English and then translated into Bahasa Malaysia through standard back-translation. The full list of items is provided in Table 2.4.

2.3.5 Statistical analysis

Data analysis was performed with SPSS version 25 (IBM Corp). Comparisons across a range of demographic categories, as well as standard symptom severity categories for depression (PHQ-9) and anxiety (GAD-7), were made between those working in essential versus non-essential services using Chi-square tests. As scores on the PHQ-9 and GAD-7 are not normally distributed, medians with interquartile range (IQR) data are presented and comparisons made with nonparametric Mann-Whitney U tests. Nonparametric Kendall's Tau correlations are used to test for correlations between discrete BCAPS item scores, PHQ-9 total scores, and GAD-7 total scores. Log-linked gamma generalised linear model analysis is then used to determine the relationship between the significant factors and the severity of depression and anxiety when controlling for potential confounds.

2.4 Findings

2.4.1 Demographic characteristics

Of the total 177 participants who completed the survey, 73 (41.2%) were essential service workers and 104 (58.8%) non-essential service workers (see Tables 2.1 and 2.2). Half (49.3%) of essential service workers were employed in transportation. The second largest number worked in the area of healthcare and medical (14%), followed by banking and finance (6.2%) and port, dock, and airport services (4.1%). Of those in non-essential services, 26.9% were in teaching and academia, 26% in managerial and executive roles, 23.1% in service and guidance (e.g. consulting) and 15.4% in administrative job categories (see Table 2.2 for complete listing). Essential and non-essential subgroups did not differ by gender, age range, ethnicity, or marital status. However, significantly fewer of those working in essential services than those in non-essential services had an educational attainment level above undergraduate level (13.7% vs 46.2, $p < 0.001$).

2.4.2 Prevalence of psychological distress

Across the entire sample ($n = 177$) the proportion of respondents scoring in the clinical range for depression (14.1%) and anxiety (12.4%) were somewhat higher than previous figures for Malaysia (e.g. 12.1% for depression [Sherina et al., 2012] and 7.8% for anxiety [Sherina et al., 2012]). See Table 2.1.

Table 2.1 Severity categories of depression and anxiety symptoms for total sample, and essential versus non-essential service subgroups with comparison of proportion above clinical cut-off

Severity category	Total, No. (%)	Essential service	Non-essential service	p value
Overall	177 (100)	73 (41.2)	104 (58.80)	
Sex				
Male	60 (34.5)	23 (32.4)	37 (35.9)	
Female	113 (64.9)	48 (67.6)	65 (63.1)	
Other	1 (0.6)	0 (0.0)	1 (1.0)	0.62
Age, years				
18–25	25 (14.2)	13 (17.8)	12 (11.7)	
26–30	42 (23.9)	22 (30.1)	20 (19.4)	
31–40	54 (30.7)	19 (26.0)	35 (34.0)	
>40	55 (31.3)	19 (26.0)	36 (35.0)	0.16
Ethnicity				
Malay	36 (20.3)	20 (27.4)	16 (15.4)	
Chinese	83 (46.9)	35 (47.9)	48 (46.2)	
Indian	39 (22.0)	13 (17.8)	26 (25.0)	
Other	19 (10.7)	5 (6.8)	14 (13.5)	0.12
Marital status				
Unmarried	87 (49.2)	35 (47.9)	52 (50.0)	
Married[a]	90 (50.8)	38 (52.1)	52 (50.0)	0.45
Education level				
<=Undergraduate	119 (67.2)	63 (86.3)	56 (53.8)	
=>Postgraduate	58 (32.8)	10 (13.7)	48 (46.2)	0.001
PHQ9, depression symptoms				
Below clinical cut-off (<10)	152 (85.9)	64 (87.7)	88 (84.6)	
Above clinical cut-off (=>10)	25 (14.1)	9 (12.3)	16 (15.4)	0.37
GAD7, anxiety symptoms				
Below clinical cut-off (<10)	155 (78.6)	66 (90.4)	7 (9.6)	
Above clinical cut-off (=>10)	22 (12.4)	7 (9.6)	15 (14.4)	0.24

[a] Married category includes one widowed participant.

There were no significant differences in proportion scoring in the clinical range between those working in an essential and non-essential service (depression: essential service 12.3% vs non-essential service 15.4%, $\chi^2 = 0.330$, $p = 0.37$; anxiety: essential service 9.6% vs non-essential service 14.4%, $\chi^2 = 0.921$, $p = 0.24$).

2.4.3 Severity of psychological distress

The overall median (IQR) scores for depression on the PHQ-9 was 3.0 (1.0–7.0) with no significant difference between essential and non-essential

Table 2.2 Service area for essential service workers ($n = 73$) and job category non-essential service workers ($n = 104$)

	n	%
Essential Service Area		
Transport by land, water, or air	36	49.3
Healthcare and medical	14	19.2
Banking and finance	5	6.2
Port, dock, and airport services	3	4.1
E-commerce	2	2.7
Hotels and accommodations	2	2.7
Production, refining, storage, supply of fuel	2	2.7
Water	1	1.4
Food supply	1	1.4
Customs	1	1.4
Any services or works determined by the Minister as essential or critical to public health safety	6	8.2
Non-Essential Service Job Category		
Teaching and academia	28	26.9
Managerial and executive	27	26.0
Service and guidance (e.g. consultant)	24	23.1
Administration	16	15.4
Technician and engineering	4	3.8
Other	2	1.9

service workers (3.0 [0.0–6.0] vs 3.0 [1.0–7.0]; $p = 0.35$), consistent with results for symptom severity (see Table 2.3). Likewise, the overall median (IQR) score for anxiety on the GAD-7 was 2.0 (0.0–6.0) with no significant difference between subgroups (2.0 [0.0–5.0] vs 3 [0.0–6.0]; $p = 0.12$). Given the lack of association between essential/non-essential service employment and either depression or anxiety symptom scores, subsequent analyses included all participants as a single group.

Table 2.3 Scores of depression and anxiety for total sample and subgroups

Scale	Total score, median (IQR)	Essential service	Non-essential service	p value
PHQ9, Depression symptoms	3.0 (1.0–7.0)	3.0 (0.0–.0)	3.0 (1.0–7.0)	0.35
GAD7, Anxiety symptoms	2.0 (0.0–6.0)	2.0 (0.0–5.0)	3.0 (0.0–6.0)	0.12

2.4.4 Behaviours and concerns and psychological distress scores

Participants tended to score higher in the PHQ-9 rating scale when they reported having more close contact with unfamiliar people ($r = 0.15$, $p = 0.048$) or with individuals confirmed to be contagious ($r = 0.23$, $p = 0.002$). Depression levels on the PHQ-9 also tended to be higher among those indicating concerns about lack of workplace support ($r = 0.21$, $p = 0.007$), uncertainty about how the pandemic threat will progress ($r = 0.32$, $p < 0.001$), uncertainty about the medical response to the pandemic ($r = 0.18$, $p = 0.02$), others perceiving them as 'contagious' ($r = 0.18$, $p = 0.02$), hostility from members of the public ($r = 0.19$, $p = 0.01$), overwhelming workload ($r = 0.34$, $p < 0.001$) and lack of time with family ($r = 0.30$, $p < 0.001$). Log-linked gamma generalised linear model analysis was then performed to further investigate the relationship between the significant variables and depression scores. The analysis showed that among the nine variables found to correlate with depressive symptoms in bivariate analysis, only item 11, *uncertainty about how the pandemic threat will progress*, made a statistically significant contribution to the prediction ($B = 0.114$, $p < 0.01$) (see Tables 2.4 and 2.5).

Those who reported having greater contact with individuals confirmed to be contagious were more likely to indicate higher levels of anxiety on the GAD-7 ($r = 0.19$, $p = 0.02$). Elevated anxiety was also higher among those reporting greater concerns about uncertainty about how the pandemic threat will progress ($r = 0.27$, $p < 0.001$), overwhelming workload ($r = 0.27$, $p < 0.001$) and lack of time with family ($r = 0.25$, $p = 0.001$). Again, log-linked gamma generalised linear model analysis was performed to further investigate the relationship between the significant variables and anxiety scores. Three out of the four items: item 2; *have contact with individuals confirmed to be contagious* ($B = 0.093$, $p < 0.05$), item 11; *uncertainty about how the pandemic threat will progress* ($B = 0.1$, $p < 0.01$) and item 16; *lack of time for family* ($B = 0.053$, $p < 0.05$) remained statistically significant predictors (see Tables 2.4 and 2.5).

2.5 Conclusion

2.5.1 Elevated psychological distress across the workforce

The Working Amidst Pandemic (WAP) Survey was developed to investigate psychological distress across the workforce, particularly those in essential services, and identify related behaviours and concerns around the

Table 2.4 Correlations between Behaviours and Concerns Amidst Pandemic Scale (BCAPS) variables and indicators of psychological distress scores (PHQ-9 for depression and GAD-7 for anxiety) ($n = 173$)

BCAPS variable	PHQ-9	GAD-7
During this period, for work purposes I:		
1 am in close contact with unfamiliar people	0.15[b]	0.10
2 have contact with individuals confirmed to be contagious	0.23[a]	0.19[b]
3 am at risk of being infected	0.13	0.08
4 take precautions to reduce risk of infection	−0.07	−0.05
5 am confident that my behaviours reduce the risk of infection	0.07	0.01
During this period, I have been concerned about:		
6 the spread of the virus generally	−0.001	0.001
7 becoming infected myself	0.08	0.04
8 led ones becoming infected	0.07	0.03
9 lack of workplace support	0.21[a]	0.10
10 lack of adequate personal protective equipment	0.16	0.05
11 uncertainty about how the pandemic threat will progress	0.32[a]	0.27[a]
12 uncertainty about the medical response to the pandemic	0.18[b]	0.09
13 others perceiving me as 'contagious'	0.18[b]	0.06
14 hostility from members of the public	0.19[b]	0.07
15 overwhelming workload	0.34[a]	0.27[a]
16 lack of time for family	0.30[a]	0.25[a]

[a] $p < 0.01$
[b] $p < 0.05$.

emerging and ongoing COVID-19 pandemic. The resulting data provides some support for the prediction that psychological distress is elevated, and that this is associated with pandemic-related concerns. However, this elevation in depression and anxiety scores appears to be similar across the workforce with no association found between working in an essential service and psychological distress. Arguably, the most striking finding is the role played by *uncertainty about how the pandemic threat will progress* in predicting both depression and anxiety scores.

Prevalence data for depression in Malaysia is relatively scarce and with wide-ranging figures previously found (e.g. Ng, 2014 for depression). However, despite limited baselines against which to make comparison, the findings in the current study of 14.1% is marginally higher than the figure of 12.1% from a pre-pandemic study employing the PHQ-9 by Sherina

Table 2.5 Summary of log-linked gamma generalised linear model for BCAPS
variables predicting psychological distress scores (PHQ-9 for depression
and GAD-7 for anxiety) (*n* = 173)

	Coefficient B	
BCAPS variable	*PHQ-9*	*GAD-7*
1. Am in close contact with unfamiliar people	0.011	–
2. Have contact with individuals confirmed to be contagious	0.080	0.093[b]
9. Lack of workplace support	0.010	–
11. Uncertainty about how the pandemic threat will progress	0.114[a]	0.100[a]
12. Uncertainty about the medical response to the pandemic	−0.046	–
13. Others perceiving me as 'contagious'	0.018	–
14. Hostility from members of the public	−0.009	–
15. Overwhelming workload	0.022	0.011
16. Lack of time for family	0.038	0.053[b]

[a] $p < 0.01$.
[b] $p < 0.05$.

et al. (2012), and almost identical to the 14.3% reported in Chew et al.'s
(2020) multi-country comparison study focusing only on healthcare workers. Thus, while it is unclear why depression symptom levels appear to
be somewhat elevated generally–irrespective of the pandemic and employment in an essential service–the high levels among Malaysian workers war-
rant further attention. In the case of depression, the generally high scores
might provide one explanation as to why there is no difference between
those in essential and non-essential services.

A more apparent difference emerged between previously identified levels
of clinically significant anxiety among Malaysians (e.g. 7.8%, Sherina et al.,
2012; 8.2%, Kader Maideen et al., 2015) and that for the present study.
While markedly higher, this figure of 12.4% across both essential and
non-essential workers during the pandemic, is lower than the 14.9% found
for Malaysian healthcare workers in Chew et al.'s (2020) study. However,
as with scores for depression symptoms, no association was found between
essential and non-essential services workers and anxiety symptoms in the
current study.

The lack of association between working in an essential service and elevated psychological distress is contrary to expectation, as well as Toh et al.'s
(2021) finding that those in non-healthcare essential services reported
significantly higher levels of depression and anxiety than those in non-
essential service roles. While the sample in the study reported here included

just 14 healthcare workers, thus not allowing for comparisons between essential service healthcare and non-healthcare subtypes, a forthcoming publication with an additional sample of healthcare workers will include this analysis. However, the lack of specificity of job role within essential service areas must be considered an important limitation of the present study and it is possible that participants did not have greater risk exposure than those working in non-essential services. Future research should include a more fine-grained examination of essential service workers measuring, or at least documenting, their degree of risk exposure.

2.5.2 Uncertainty, contact and psychological distress

Uncertainty about how the pandemic threat will progress was the only pandemic-related concern contributing significantly to both depression and anxiety symptom scores and this is of theoretical and practical interest. This is consistent with the findings from a cross-sectional survey conducted during the first UK lockdown in late April 2020 which found intolerance of uncertainty to be predictive of anxiety and depression (Rettie and Daniels, 2020), and the survey of Malaysians conducted around the same time cited in "Introduction" section (Mahmud et al., 2020).

Rutter et al. (2020) have emphasised that uncertainty is inevitable during pandemics and, within a complex informational climate where 'uncontested facts tend to be elusive', the importance of accepting that uncertainties cannot be resolved. An emerging body of research addresses uncertainty distress in the context of COVID-19 explicitly, exploring for example ways in which threat and uncertainty are separable in anxiety, and suggesting therapeutic techniques such as challenging beliefs, increasing tolerance of uncertainty, and supporting selective access to types of pandemic-related information (Freeston at al., 2020). Moreover, intolerance of uncertainty has been identified as a potential transdiagnostic dispositional risk factor (Carleton et al., 2012), consistent with the predictive utility observed across anxiety and depression in the current study.

Working in close contact with positive cases also appears to have a bearing on anxiety. That endorsement of *have contact with individuals confirmed to be contagious* was found to predict anxiety is consistent with the findings of Lai et al.'s (2020) study among healthcare workers in China. Lai et al.'s (2020) results, which informed the development of the present study, indicated that those working most directly with infected patients, and in places closest to concentrations of infection (i.e. Wuhan), reported the highest levels of anxiety and depression. A forthcoming publication including a sample of Malaysian healthcare workers will further examine the relative predictive value of this variable.

Finally, the finding that being concerned about *lack of time for family* during the pandemic period is associated with elevated anxiety appears to be a novel one. However, further research is needed to determine if the association is linked to—or occurs independently of—working amidst pandemic. Moreover, if this concern does reflect an objective reduction in time available to dedicate to family because of the pandemic, it should be examined differently for those working from home and those who have continued in their place of work. While it suggests a possible paradox in the shift to working from home—wherein time reclaimed from commutes and proximity to family during working hours is accompanied by a *decrease* in available family time—it might be an indication of extra time burden through newly introduced SOPs, especially for those in essential service roles continuing with 'business as usual'.

2.5.3 *Limitations of the study*

The study presented in this chapter had a number of limitations. Perhaps most notably, while data were collected during the early phase of the pandemic mapping onto findings from other cited studies, the number of cases during that time between May and August were extremely low (often in single digits for new daily cases) with the first real wave starting in September. At the same time, the findings of elevated psychological distress remain of interest whether it be despite or potentially as a result of the low levels of infection (i.e. anxiety around an unknown/impending threat). Comparisons to data collected during the main waves of infection, with daily rates in the thousands, are called for.

Specific concerns around the pandemic were determined with discrete questions created for the purposes of this study without thorough content validation. Systematic development of multi-item scales to gage key concerns, and/or validation of the single items used, would allow for greater confidence in the results.

Moreover, psychological distress was based entirely on brief self-report measures. While these are widely used reliable and valid instruments, the study would have been strengthened with the inclusion of diagnostic interview-based data. Furthermore, categorisation into essential and non-essential workers was also based on unverified self-report which may have been knowingly or unwittingly inaccurate.

Finally, while the sample allowed for comparisons between the two main groups, it did not allow for comparisons of subgroups of essential service workers. Finer analyses might well reveal that working in some services are associated with greater risk than others.

2.5.4 Summary

On balance, the study findings reported here present a relatively low-resolution snapshot of psychological distress across the workforce during the early period of COVID-19 spread in Malaysia. The juxtaposition of relatively high levels of anxiety and depression, found in the current study consistent with data reported elsewhere, at a time when infection rates were actually very low is striking. What appears to be the critical vulnerability factor of concerns about uncertainty as to how the pandemic threat will continue provides a useful indication for supporting individual and societal level psychological distress.

Practical suggestions

Public health messaging, at a national, local, and organisational level, acknowledging the role of uncertainty in psychological distress suggests itself as an upstream strategy to mitigate anxiety and depression. For example, employers might provide staff with reassurance on matters with relative predictability (such as continued operations) whilst also offering a supportive acknowledgement and flexible response to uncertainty (such as disruptions to work-life balance through pandemic-related changes to family/household matters like childcare). Integration of related techniques into psychological interventions for those presenting to services should be considered.

Acknowledgement

We thank Dr Nor Hayati Binti Ali (Department of Psychiatry and Mental Health, Selayang Hospital), Dr Muhammad Haniff Bin Abdullah (Department of Psychiatry and Mental Health, Selayang Hospital), Mr Tamil Selvan Ramis (HELP University) Mr. Rubendev Singh Dhillon (Malaysian Mental Health Association), and Dr Aini Hamid (University of Nottingham Malaysia) for their contributions to the development and implementation of this research. We also extend our gratitude to the many organisations and individuals who supported recruitment and participated in the study.

Note

1. Malaysian Federal Government Gazette 'Prevention and Control of Infectious Diseases (Measures within the Affected Local Areas) Regulations 2020' issued March 18, 2020 to cover the period of Movement Control Order (MCO).

References

Carleton, R. N., Mulvogue, M. K., Thibodeau, M. A., McCabe, R. E., Antony, M. M., & Asmundson, G. J. (2012). Increasingly certain about uncertainty: Intolerance of uncertainty across anxiety and depression. *Journal of Anxiety Disorders*, 26, 468–479. https://doi.org/10.1016/j.janxdis.2012.01.011.

Chew, N., Ngiam, J. N., Tan, B. Y., Tham, S. M., Tan, C. Y., Jing, M., Sagayanathan, R., Chen, J. T., Wong, L., Ahmad, A., Khan, F. A., Marmin, M., Hassan, F. B., Sharon, T. M., Lim, C. H., Mohaini, M., Danuaji, R., Nguyen, T. H., Tsivgoulis, G., Tsiodras, S., & Sharma, V. K. (2020). Asian-Pacific perspective on the psychological well-being of healthcare workers during the evolution of the COVID-19 pandemic. *BJPsych open*, 6(6), e116. https://doi.org/10.1192/bjo.2020.98

Freeston, M., Tiplady, A., Mawn, L., Bottesi, G., & Thwaites, S. (2020). Towards a model of uncertainty distress in the context of coronavirus (COVID-19). *The Cognitive Behaviour Therapist*, 13, E31. doi:10.1017/S1754470X2000029X

Giorgi, G., Lecca, L. I., Alessio, F., Finstad, G. L., Bondanini, G., Lulli, L. G., Arcangeli, G., & Mucci, N. (2020). COVID-19-related mental health effects in the workplace: A narrative review. *International journal of environmental research and public health*, 17(21), 7857.

Hyland, P., Shevlin, M., McBride, O., Murphy, J., Karatzias, T., Bentall, R. P., Martinez, A., & Vallières, F. (2020). Anxiety and depression in the Republic of Ireland during the COVID-19 pandemic. *Acta psychiatrica Scandinavica*, 142(3), 249–256. https://doi.org/10.1111/acps.13219

Kader Maideen, S. F., Sidik, S. M., Rampal, L., & Mukhtar, F. (2014). Prevalence, associated factors and predictors of depression among adults in the community of Selangor, Malaysia. *PloS One*, 9(4), e95395. https://doi.org/10.1371/journal.pone.0095395

Kniffin, K. M., Narayanan, J., Anseel, F., Antonakis, J., Ashford, S. P., Bakker, A. B., Bamberger, P., Bapuji, H., Bhave, D. P., Choi, V. K., Creary, S. J., Demerouti, E., Flynn, F. J., Gelfand, M. J., Greer, L. L., Johns, G., Kesebir, S., Klein, P. G., Lee, S. Y., ... Vugt, M. v. (2021). COVID-19 and the workplace: Implications, issues, and insights for future research and action. *American Psychologist*, 76(1), 63–77. https://doi.org/10.1037/amp0000716

Kroenke, K., Spitzer, R. L., & Williams, J. B. W. (2001). The PHQ-9: Validity of a brief depression severity measure. *Journal of General Internal Medicine*, 16(9), 606–613. doi:10.1046/j.1525-1497.2001.016009606.x

Lai, J., Ma, S., Wang, Y., Cai, Z., Hu, J., Wei, N., Wu, J., Du, H., Chen, T., Li, R., Tan, H., Kang, L., Yao, L., Huang, M., Wang, H., Wang, G., Liu, Z., & Hu, S. (2020). Factors associated with mental health outcomes among health care workers exposed to coronavirus disease 2019. *JAMA network open*, 3(3), e203976. https://doi.org/10.1001/jamanetworkopen.2020.3976

Li, J., Yang, Z., Qiu, H., Wang, Y., Jian, L., Ji, J., & Li, K. (2020). Anxiety and depression among general population in China at the peak of the COVID-19 epidemic. *World Psychiatry: Official Journal of the World Psychiatric Association (WPA)*, 19(2), 249–250. https://doi.org/10.1002/wps.20758

Mahmud, Z., Abdul Rahim, R., Zainan Abidin, A. W., & Abdullah, N. N. N. (2020). Mental and emotional wellbeing during the COVID-19 pandemic: The unprecedented Malaysian experience. *Current Psychiatry Research and Reviews*, 16(4). https://doi.org/10.2174/2666082216666201013153842

Malaysian Federal Government Gazette 'Prevention and Control of Infectious Diseases (Measures within the Affected Local Areas) Regulations 2020'. Issued 18 March 2020. http://www.federalgazette.agc.gov.my/outputp/pua_20200318_PUA91_2020.pdf

Mehta, S., Machado, F., Kwizera, A., Papazian, L., Moss, M., Azoulay, É, & Herridge, M. (2021). COVID-19: A heavy toll on health-care workers. *The Lancet. Respiratory Medicine*, 9(3), 226–228. https://doi.org/10.1016/S2213-2600(21)00068-0

Ng, C. G. (2014). A review of depression research in Malaysia. *The Medical Journal of Malaysia*, 69(Supplement A), 42–45.

Rettie, H., & Daniels, J. (2020). Coping and tolerance of uncertainty: Predictors and mediators of mental health during the COVID-19 pandemic. *American Psychologist*. Advance online publication. http://dx.doi.org/10.1037/amp0000710

Roslan, N. S., Yusoff, M. S. B., Asrenee, A. R., & Morgan, K. (2021). Burnout prevalence and its associated factors among Malaysian healthcare workers during COVID-19 pandemic: An embedded mixed-method study. *Healthcare*, 9(1), 90. doi:10.3390/healthcare9010090

Rutter, H., Wolpert, M., & Greenhalgh, T. (2020). Managing uncertainty in the covid-19 era *BMJ*, 370, m3349. https://www.bmj.com/content/bmj/370/bmj.m3349.full.pdf

Shah, A., Safri, S., Thevadas, R., Noordin, N. K., Rahman, A. A., Sekawi, Z., Ideris, A., & Sultan, M. (2020). COVID-19 outbreak in Malaysia: Actions taken by the Malaysian government. *International Journal of Infectious Diseases: IJID: Official Publication of the International Society for Infectious Diseases*, 97, 108–116. https://doi.org/10.1016/j.ijid.2020.05.093

Sheraton, M., Deo, N., Dutt, T., Surani, S., Hall-Flavin, D., & Kashyap, R. (2020). Psychological effects of the COVID 19 pandemic on healthcare workers globally: A systematic review. *Psychiatry research*, 292, 113360. https://doi.org/10.1016/j.psychres.2020.113360

Sherina M. S., Arroll, B., & Goodyear-Smith, F. (2012). Criterion validity of the PHQ-9 (Malay version) in a primary care clinic in Malaysia. *The Medical Journal of Malaysia*, 67(3), 309–315.

Shevlin, M., McBride, O., Murphy, J., Miller, J. G., Hartman, T. K., Levita, L., Mason, L., Martinez, A. P., McKay, R., Stocks, T., Bennett, K. M., Hyland, P., Karatzias, T., & Bentall, R. P. (2020). Anxiety, depression, traumatic stress and COVID-19-related anxiety in the UK general population during the COVID-19 pandemic. *BJPsych Open*, 6(6), e125. https://doi.org/10.1192/bjo.2020.109

Sidik, S. M., Arroll, B., & Goodyear-Smith, F. (2012). Validation of the GAD-7 (Malay version) among women attending a primary care clinic in Malaysia. *Journal of Primary Health Care*, 4(1), 5–11. doi:10.1071/HC12005

Spitzer, R. L., Kroenke, K., Williams, J. B. W., & Löwe, B. (2006). A brief measure for assessing generalized anxiety disorder: The GAD-7. *Archives of Internal Medicine, 166*(10), 1092–1097. doi:10.1001/archinte.166.10.1092

Tan, B., Chew, N., Lee, G., Jing, M., Goh, Y., Yeo, L., Zhang, K., Chin, H. K., Ahmad, A., Khan, F. A., Shanmugam, G. N., Chan, B., Sunny, S., Chandra, B., Ong, J., Paliwal, P. R., Wong, L., Sagayanathan, R., Chen, J. T., Ng, A., & Sharma, V. K. (2020). Psychological impact of the COVID-19 pandemic on health care workers in Singapore. *Annals of Internal Medicine, 173*(4), 317–320. https://doi.org/10.7326/M20-1083

The Lancet. (2020). The plight of essential workers during the COVID-19 pandemic. *Lancet (London, England), 395*(10237), 1587. https://doi.org/10.1016/S0140-6736(20)31200-9

Toh, W. L., Meyer, D., Phillipou, A., Tan, E. J., Van Rheenen, T. E., Neill, E., et al. (2021). Mental health status of healthcare versus other essential workers in Australia amidst the COVID-19 pandemic: Initial results from the collate project. *Psychiatry Research, 298*, 113822. doi: 10.1016/j.psychres.2021.113822

Valiente, C., Contreras, A., Peinado, V., Trucharte, A., Martínez, A., & Vázquez, C. (2021). Psychological adjustment in Spain during the COVID-19 pandemic: Positive and negative mental health outcomes in the general population. *The Spanish Journal of Psychology, 24*, E8. doi:10.1017/SJP.2021.7

Xiao, Y., Becerik-Gerber, B., Lucas, G., & Roll, S. C. (2021). Impacts of working from home during COVID-19 pandemic on physical and mental well-being of office workstation users. *Journal of Occupational and Environmental Medicine, 63*(3), 181–190. https://doi.org/10.1097/JOM.0000000000002097

Section II
Predictors of distress and mental health

3 Psychosocial and demographic predictors of mental health and distress

Hasse De Meyer, Farihin Ufiya, & Siew Li Ng

3.1 Introduction

The spread of the COVID-19 pandemic was first documented in 2019 in Wuhan City, China. By April 2020, over 200 countries were affected by the virus. Due to the lack of human immunity and the explosive spread of COVID-19, policy makers and virologists focused on reducing human transmission through social distancing to restrain the debilitating and mortal consequences. A restriction in movement was therefore enforced in Malaysia starting on March 18, 2020 (Movement Control Order, MCO; Shah et al., 2020) and led to extended social distancing.

The impact of a pandemic, however, goes beyond the direct medical consequences. Earlier pandemics like SARS and Ebola disrupted essential services such as education, transport and tourism, and challenged the economy and healthcare systems (WHO, 2018). During the first MCO, a special survey from the Department of Statistics Malaysia reported that 67.80% of businesses had no sales or revenue. Further, the overall GDP dropped by 17.10% in the second quartile of 2020, and the country's existing unemployment crisis was exacerbated with a monthly increase of 10,000 unemployed individuals (Zhou et al., 2021). The global economy faced historical challenges leading to a global recession (e.g. increased unemployment ratio), disproportionately affecting low to middle income countries, such as Malaysia (Vassall et al., 2020). Such financial crises come with an increase in substance abuse, depression and anxiety, and prolonged unemployment is associated with increased suicide rates (Classen & Dunn, 2012).

The pandemic affects mental health, where increased anxiety, depression and post-traumatic stress symptoms are already evidenced in most countries (Xiong et al., 2020). In just the first seven days of the MCO, a non-profit suicide hotline (Befrienders) reported a 13% increase in calls (News Straits Times, 2020) along with 43,078 calls to the COVID-19 mental health hotline as of 1 December 2020 (House of Senate, 2020).

DOI: 10.4324/9781003178576-5

Unfortunately, insufficient resources were made available to address the impact on mental health, as these problems are often neglected. Especially in countries such as Malaysia where access to mental health is less prioritized and well-established due to more precedent matters such as physical healthcare and economics, the demand for help in this area is higher than the services available (Chong et al., 2013). This is evident as guidelines for mental health and psychosocial support following the MCO were only released by the Ministry of Health (MOH) two months after the first outbreak in Malaysia (MOH, 2021).

3.2 Literature review

3.2.1 Predictors of mental health

In Malaysia, mental health is defined as "the capacity of the individual, the group and environment to affective and relational abilities, towards the achievement of individual and collective goals consistent with justice" (MOH, 2021). The strong emphasis on the collective nature in the definition refers to its multi-cultural society (67.40% Malays; 24.60% Chinese and 7.30% Indians) (Institute for Public Health, 2020). In collectivistic cultures, social networks are of the utmost importance and associated with interdependence on each other. When comparing individualistic and collectivist cultures, research suggests that feelings of loneliness are likely to be higher and sensitivity to social isolation is stronger in collectivistic cultures (Swader, 2019). Many studies conducted during COVID-19 have found exacerbated levels of loneliness and internalizing symptoms (Xiong et al., 2020), which are likely due to prolonged physical isolation and uncertainties posed during the pandemic. Hence, people from collectivistic countries such as Malaysia may fare worse in response to physical distancing measures.

While it can be suggested that the use of social media platforms mitigates feelings of loneliness and social distancing during a stay-at-home order, several studies show that increased exposure to social media is associated with internalising disorders during COVID-19 (Xiong et al., 2020). Even during non-pandemic times, increased mental health issues have often been linked to social media which is attributed to social comparisons with others and social support quality (e.g. Keles et al., 2020). In addition to social media use, a variety of socio-demographic variables such as age, female gender, and income level, as well as stressors such as work stress and comorbidity are often linked to mental health and well-being outcomes (Chan et al., 2021; Kader Maideen et al., 2015). Some of these variables have already been identified to be risk factors of adverse mental health during the COVID-19 pandemic (e.g. younger age, female gender, unemployment; Xiong et al., 2020). Other factors that were found to increase risk of mental distress include presence of chronic or psychiatric illness, being single or separated, low social support, loneliness and increased social media use (Rens et al., 2021; Wang et al., 2021; Xiong et al., 2020). This pattern of data is observed across countries, which begs the question—are Malaysian residents responding similarly to the pandemic, especially in terms of mental health outcomes and risk and protective factors?

3.2.2 Mental health in Malaysia

Pertaining to mental illness, Malaysians have a strong devotion to more traditional ethnic-specific belief systems, e.g. spirit possession or social punishment in Malay culture, the imbalance of Yin and Yang in Chinese culture, and the imbalance of Dharma, Kama, Artha and Moksha in Indian culture (Haque, 2005). They display lower levels of mental health knowledge, but also stigmatizing beliefs towards mental health issues, even in staff providing mental health services (Munawar et al., 2021). Nevertheless, Malaysia does not escape the global surge of mental health difficulties, even before the pandemic. In the past decade (1996–2016), the prevalence of mental health issues has tripled (10.70% vs 29.20%) with anxiety and depressive disorders as the main contributors leading to disability (Chua, 2020; Institute for Public Health, 2015).

Despite an average worldwide prevalence of mental health issues in Malaysia, reaching out to professional help for mental health difficulties often remains associated with feelings of shame both for the individual and their family with a potential risk of social exclusion (Chong et al., 2013). Even when mental health services are considered, access is limited due to the large disparity between fees in private and public mental health services, as well as uneven distribution of these services across different states, particularly lacking in rural areas (Lim, 2018). This is pertinent given the higher rates of mental illness in rural areas and those of lower socioeconomic status (Institute for Public Health, 2020).

Given Malaysia's distinctive cultural system, socioeconomic environment and implementation of physical distancing measures, it is essential to know how Malaysians were affected given the prolonged MCO. The following sections report a study done during the COVID-19 pandemic, examining various aspects of mental health, including psychological well-being, internalising symptoms (i.e., depression, anxiety and stress) and levels of loneliness and social support.

3.3 Method

3.3.1 Sample

A total of 1,234 participants, aged 18–65 years, participated in the study. The criteria for selection were: (1) residing in Malaysia, (2) at least 18 years old and (3) able to read and understand English or Bahasa Malaysia.

3.3.2 Data collection and measures

Data collection was initiated on May 11, 2020 at the start of the Conditional MCO (CMCO) for 2.5 weeks. The survey was advertised through social media and the researchers' network. Ethical approval from HELP University was obtained. Participants first provided informed consent, and upon completing the survey, were eligible to win a 50 Malaysian Ringgit (MYR) voucher.

The following data was collected through Qualtrics.com:

1 Demographic variables such as household composition, nationality, lodging, (change in) income and employment, education, etc.
2 Social media use was categorized in three levels (less than 3 hours, between 3 to 6 hours, more than 6 hours). The change from conventional daily use to current daily use was operationalized in three categories: no increase, a small increase (shift of one category) and large increase (shift of two categories).
3 Loneliness was measured using a modification of the UCLA 3-item Loneliness scale (Rens et al., 2021) on a 4-point Likert scale. The differentiation between levels of loneliness was based upon a cut-off score (score ≥ 8, lonely; score < 8, not lonely).
4 The 3-item Oslo Social Support Scale (OSSS-3; Dalgard, 1996) was utilized to measure social support. Three categories were derived from the sum score: poor support (3–8), moderate support (9–11) and strong support (12–14) (Kocalevent et al., 2018).

3.3.3 Outcome measures

Depressive, anxiety and stress symptoms were measured using the Depression Anxiety Stress Scales (DASS-21; Lovibond & Lovibond, 1995). These symptoms were rated over the past week on a 4-point Likert scale. Total scores are multiplied by 2 for norm comparison.

Mental well-being was measured by the 12-item General Health Questionnaire (GHQ-12; Goldberg & Williams, 1988). The GHQ-scoring (i.e. 0 0 1 1) is applied leading to a sum score ranging between

0 and 12. A cut-off score of ≥ 4 was used to distinguish respondents suffering from mental distress (Lundin et al., 2017).

3.4 Findings

The outcome measures (DASS-21 and GHQ-12) were analysed using ANOVA and t-test to compare groups, as well as linear multiple and logistic regressions to predict the association between predictors and outcome variables. All the measures have good internal consistencies ranging from 0.85 to 0.95, except OSSS-3 ($a = 0.54$). This relatively low value has been attributed to its brevity (Kocalevent et al., 2018); nonetheless, interpretation of social support results should be done with caution.

As group sizes were not evenly distributed, Games-Howell post-test was used for the ANOVAs. Binary logistic regressions were used to estimate the odds of being mentally distressed (i.e. GHQ cases). The predictor-outcome relationships were expressed as crude odds ratio (COR), with corresponding 95% confidence intervals (95% CI). Those with a significant Wald test ($p < 0.05$) were included in the same model with multiple predictors, and adjusted odds ratios (AOR), with a 95% CI, were calculated. Based on the a priori hypotheses and analyses needed, a sample size of at least 570 individuals were needed to achieve a power of 0.80 for this study.

3.4.1 Sample characteristics

Only responses from those residing in Malaysia at the time of the survey were included in the analyses. Data was collected from 1,234 individuals ($M = 25.94$, $SD = 7.27$), majority of whom were female (83.60%), Malaysians (97.10%), involved in or completed a professional degree or undergraduate education (73.70%), single (59.90%), living with family/partner/flatmates (93.10%) and earning less than 4,000 MYR (82.10%). The majority completed the survey in English (88.50%). Some indicated having prior mental health services (18.20%), current chronic illness (15.60%), limited activities due to health problems (12.40%) and being exposed to COVID-19 (confirmed cases or living with confirmed cases; 0.60%). Respondents also indicated their pattern in: income level (same: 56.20%; decreased: 40.30%), workload (same: 34.50%; increased: 35.70%), and social media use (same usage: 44.20%; increased: 51.70%) (see Table 3.1).

Overall, moderate levels of depression ($M = 15.89$; $SD = 12.25$) and anxiety ($M = 10.89$; $SD = 9.70$), and mild levels of stress ($M = 15.39$; $SD = 10.65$) were reported. Close to half of the respondents experienced low social support (44.80% vs 47.20% for moderate and 8.0% for high social support) and feelings of loneliness (41.80%), and over half of those surveyed were categorized as distressed (58.20%).

Table 3.1 Demographic characteristics of respondents (Malaysian residents) (*n* = 1,234)

	Male	Female
Gender (N/%)[a]	194 (15.72)	1032 (83.63)
Age (M/SD)[a]	27.91 (8.26)	25.58 (7.03)
Education qualification (N/%)		
Low	25 (12.89)	170 (16.47)
Middle	144 (74.23)	759 (73.55)
High	23 (11.86)	96 (9.30)
Other	2 (1.03)	7 (0.68)
Occupation		
Student	67 (34.53)	448 (43.41)
Employed	107 (55.15)	440 (42.64)
Unemployed	20 (10.30)	137 (13.28)
Other	0	7 (0.68)
Relationship status[a]		
Single	118 (60.82)	618 (59.88)
Relationship/Married	69 (35.57)	393 (38.08)
Divorced/Widowed	4 (2.06)	16 (1.55)
Accommodation[a]		
Family	133 (68.56)	823 (79.75)
Flatmates/Partner	40 (20.62)	145 (14.05)
Alone	13 (6.70)	49 (4.75)
Others	5 (2.58)	10 (0.97)
Monthly income (MYR)[a]		
0-4,000	143 (73.71)	863 (83.62)
4,001-10,000	28 (14.43)	141 (13.66)
>10,001	22 (11.34)	18 (1.74)

Note: Low = Primary, Secondary school, Vocational and Pre-U/STPM; Middle = Undergraduate, Professional Degree; High = Postgraduate; MYR = Malaysian Ringgit.

[a] Missing data: Gender (*N* = 8); Age (*N* = 3, Female; *N* = 2, Male); Relationship status (*N* = 3, Male; *N* = 5, Female); Accommodation (*N* = 3, Male; *N* = 5, Female); Income (*N* = 1, Male; *N* = 10, Female).

3.4.2 Depressive, anxiety and stress levels

3.4.2.1 Demographic characteristic differences

Depressive, anxiety and stress levels were strongly related to one another (r = 0.71–0.81, $p < 0.001$), suggesting that respondents who had more depressive symptoms tend to have more stress and anxiety symptoms, and vice versa. Respondents with an individual monthly income below 2,000 MYR as compared to > 2,000 MYR, reported higher levels of depression, anxiety and stress. Age, gender, loneliness, psychiatric history and chronic illness jointly predicted depressive symptoms, $R^2 = 0.34$, $F(5, 1208) = 126.02$, $p < 0.001$; all of them but gender were significant predictors, while holding respective predictors constant. Similar results were observed for anxiety symptoms: age, gender, loneliness, psychiatric history and chronic illness jointly predicted 25.5% of variance in anxiety symptoms, $F(5, 1208) = 82.76$, $p < 0.001$. For stress, however, all predictors including gender, significantly predicted stress symptoms while holding respective predictors constant: age, gender, loneliness, psychiatric history, and chronic illness, $R^2 = 0.30$, $F(5, 1210) = 41.38$, $p < 0.001$. Living arrangements did not contribute to the outcome variables; however, very uneven groups were reported.

3.4.2.2 Impact of changes

Depressive, anxiety and stress levels were significantly different for those who had changes in income ($p < 0.01$). Specifically, those who had decreased income reported higher levels of depressive ($M = 17.60$) and anxiety symptoms ($M = 12.54$) than those who had the same ($M_{dep} = 14.85$; $M_{anx} = 9.77$) or an increased income ($M_{dep} = 11.89$; $M_{anx} = 8.76$). Respondents with decreased income ($M = 16.60$) had higher levels of stress than those without changes in income ($M = 14.56$).

Results showed that changes in workload influenced anxiety, stress and depressive symptoms ($p < 0.01$). More specifically, respondents who, because of MCO, had an increase ($M = 16.75$) or decrease in workload ($M = 16.59$) experienced higher levels of depression as compared to those whose workload remained stable ($M = 14.44$). An increase ($M_{str} = 17.19$; $M_{anx} = 12.10$) in workload leads to more stress and anxiety than those with an identical workload ($M_{str} = 13.68$; $M_{anx} = 9.52$); those with increased workload had higher stress level than those with a decrease ($M = 15.21$).

The amount of time spent on social media is a significant predictor for symptoms of depression, anxiety and stress ($p < 0.001$). Those who reported spending more than 6 hours per day on social media ($M_{dep} = 18.06$; $M_{anx} = 12.24$; $M_{str} = 16.92$) reported significantly higher depressive, anxiety and stress symptoms than those who spend 3–6 hours ($M_{dep} = 13.24$; $M_{anx} = 9.36$; $M_{str} = 13.42$) or less than 3 hours per day ($M_{dep} = 12.51$; $M_{anx} = 8.43$; $M_{str} = 13.32$). Furthermore, the extent of changes in time spent on social media since the outbreak of the pandemic also predicted stress ($p < 0.05$), where stress level was higher for respondents who reported a large increase ($M = 18.05$) compared to those who had a small increase ($M = 15.32$) and had no change ($M = 14.82$) in their social media use.

3.4.2.3 Social support

There was also a clear difference in depressive, anxiety and stress symptoms when comparing the levels of social support ($p < 0.001$). Post-hoc comparisons revealed that those with low social support had the highest depressive and stress levels ($M_{dep} = 20.06$; $M_{str} = 18.18$), followed by those with moderate social support ($M_{dep} = 13.17$; $M_{str} = 13.66$), and subsequently high social support ($M_{dep} = 8.57$; $M_{str} = 10.00$). Further, those with low social support ($M = 12.96$) experienced more anxiety symptoms compared to those with moderate ($M = 9.48$) and high social support ($M = 7.58$).

3.4.3 Mental distress

Binary logistic regression analyses showed that the following risk factors are significantly associated with being mentally distressed (GHQ $\geq$ 4): female, student or unemployed, income below 2,000 MYR, decreased income, experiencing chronic illness, history of mental health services, having limited movement due to a health problem, increased workload, large or small increase in time spent on social media, lost a job, low or moderate social support and loneliness. Being older, in a relationship, and having the same workload as before the outbreak were protective factors against being mentally distressed (see Table 3.2).

These 14 significant predictors were then included into a binary logistic regression model. Controlling the effects of the respective predictors, the adjusted odds of being mentally distressed were higher for females and those who had increased workload, having lost their job, have a large increase in time spent on social media, having had prior experience with psychological services, have low social support, and are experiencing loneliness (see Table 3.2).

3.5 Conclusion

The literature showed an ongoing increase in mental health difficulties over the past years. Combined with a low mental health literacy, a strong prejudice against those suffering from mental illness, insufficient access to mental health practitioners and facilities and a pandemic, it predisposes Malaysia to be at high risk for an unprecedented increase of mental health difficulties.

Findings show that specific demographic characteristics are associated with poorer mental health e.g. younger age, being female, lower income, presence of a chronic illness and psychiatry history and employment status.

For instance, respondents with an individual monthly income below 2,000 MYR, as compared to > 2,000 MYR, reported higher levels of depression, anxiety and stress. Such risk factors are not uncommon, and these results are consistent with past findings (e.g. Institute for Public Health, 2020; Wang et al., 2021). The impact of the pandemic and physical quarantine is highlighted in this study; many had a decrease in income, increase in workload and social media use, and a change in working conditions. Such changes are also observed in other studies (Xiong et al., 2020). Among these changes, respondents with a large increase in social media use were 2.15 times more likely to have mental distress than those with no change. Compared with those without changes to their work conditions, the chances of being mentally distressed was 4.22 times higher for those who had lost their job. Those risk factors continue to be significant even after other risk factors are controlled in the statistical analyses.

Alarming results are seen in respondents who reported experiencing low social support and loneliness. Those who perceived having low social support were 5.09 times more likely to be mentally distressed and reported the highest levels of depressive, stress, and anxiety symptoms. The risk of being mentally distressed was 7.02 times more for those who were lonely. The higher prevalence of loneliness observed in this more collectivistic sample, compared to more individualistic samples in Belgian (Rens et al., 2021) and Italian (Fiorillo et al., 2020) studies is in line with the previous research suggesting higher levels of loneliness in collectivist cultures (Swader, 2019).

The prevalence of mental distress (GHQ > 4) in the Malaysian[1] sample is far below those observed in Italian (91.2%; Fiorillo et al., 2020), and Belgian (65.49%; Rens et al., 2021); but higher compared to the UK sample (36.70%; Pierce et al., 2020b). Upon comparing lockdown effects on depression, anxiety and stress symptoms with other countries, Malaysians report high levels of internalising symptoms (e.g. Wang et al., 2021). One of the most severely impacted countries at the onset of the COVID-19 pandemic was Italy. Upon comparison with Italy, Malaysians report similar levels of stress ($M_{Malaysia} = 15.39$; $M_{Italy} = 16.30$), but higher levels of depression ($M_{Malaysia} = 15.89$; $M_{Italy} = 12.20$) and anxiety ($M_{Malaysia} = 10.89$; $M_{Italy} = 7.40$) (Fiorillo et al., 2020). Despite the different lockdown restrictions in both countries, the data shows that the pandemic has a devastating impact on Malaysians' mental health.

3.5.1 Guidelines and policies

Our findings highlight the importance of considering the mental health implications of the pandemic, which have largely been neglected in the

Table 3.2 Prevalence of mental distress and its associated odd ratio by predictor category

Predictor	% distress	COR	95% CI	p	AOR	95% CI	p
Age		0.96	0.95–0.98	0.000	0.99	0.96–1.01	0.214
Gender							
Male	46.91	1			1		
Female	60.27	1.72	1.26–2.34	0.001	1.48	1.02–2.15	0.040
Employment status							
Employed	51.55	1			1		
Unemployed	61.78	1.52	1.06–2.19	0.024	0.90	0.51–1.61	0.733
Student	63.69	1.66	1.30–2.12	0.000	0.98	0.061–1.56	0.916
Income							
≤MYR 2,000	63.01	1.71	1.35–2.16	0.000	1.39	1.02–2.15	0.157
>MYR 2,000	50.22	1			1		
Income change							
Increase	37.84	1			1		
No change	53.77	1.93	0.98–3.81	0.059	1.50	0.67–3.39	0.329
Decrease	65.85	3.13	1.57–6.24	0.001	2.15	0.93–4.96	0.074
Work condition change							
No change	52.73	1			1		
More time at work	46.99	0.78	0.48–1.28	0.331	0.70	0.36–1.35	0.286
More time at home	56.10	1.13	0.84–1.51	0.418	1.15	0.78–1.71	0.483
Work stoppage	59.49	1.30	0.78–2.16	0.312	0.89	0.48–1.70	0.730
Lost my job	82.43	4.22	2.22–8.02	0.000	3.28	1.52–7.40	0.003
Other	66.85	1.75	1.19–2.59	0.005	1.29	0.78–2.04	0.303
Workload change							
Decrease	58.77	1			1		
No change	47.41	0.64	0.49–0.85	0.002	0.89	0.62–1.28	0.539
Increase	68.26	1.52	1.14–2.03	0.005	2.41	1.64–3.55	0.000
Relationship status							
Not in a relationship	61.38	1			1		
In a relationship	52.81	0.70	0.56–0.89	0.003	0.98	0.72–1.32	0.873
Psychiatry history							
No	54.17	1			1		
Yes	75.45	2.60	1.87–3.61	0.000	2.02	1.34–3.04	0.001
Chronic illness							
No	56.18	1			1		
Yes	67.73	1.65	1.19–2.29	0.003	0.85	0.55–1.32	0.471
Limited mobility							
No	56.15	1			1		
Yes	70.86	1.94	1.34–2.81	0.000	1.58	0.98–2.54	0.060
Loneliness							
No	40.76	1			1		
Yes	82.58	7.02	5.35–9.23	0.000	5.17	3.80–7.05	0.000
Social media use							
No increase	53.43	1			1		
Small increase	60.89	1.36	1.07–1.73	0.014	2.23	1.32–3.74	0.070
Large increase	71.19	2.15	1.40–3.31	0.001	1.31	0.98–1.76	0.003

(*Continued*)

Table 3.2 Prevalence of mental distress and its associated odd ratio by predictor category (*Continued*)

Predictor	% distress	COR	95% CI	p	AOR	95% CI	p
Social support							
High	33.67	1			1		
Moderate	49.40	1.96	1.25–3.07	0.003	1.37	0.81–2.33	0.002
Low	71.77	5.09	3.22–8.04	0.000	2.32	1.35–4.00	0.000

Abbreviations: AOR, adjusted odds ratio; 95% CI, 95% confidence interval; COR, crude odds ratio.

current public health discourse in Malaysia. Given the immense psychological impact involved, we encourage the inclusion of the evidence-based and up-to-date mental health responses in the primary guideline for future crises.

Beyond these guidelines, MOH should also publish a strategic and comprehensive mitigation plan for the impending post-COVID-19 mental health crisis, which may involve training as mental health practitioners are worryingly limited, e.g. only 15 clinical psychologists were employed in the entire public health sector in 2018, and merely 1 psychiatrist is available per 100,000 population (APA recommended ratio: 1:10,000; Relate Mental Health Malaysia, 2020). With regards to adequate training, MOH's well-intended mitigation efforts, which primarily involve the hiring and deployment of counsellors with minimal Bachelor's degrees, leave a lot to be desired. Besides training, there needs to be a redistribution of the mental health workforce across different states to address the limited access in rural areas.

Mental health researchers and practitioners should be consulted in said mitigation plan. Furthermore, the interventions proposed should be subsequently audited for impact and efficacy, given that the lack of post-implementation auditing is a recurring problem in Malaysia's mental health policies (Yap et al., 2020).

As discussed earlier, access to mental health services is particularly limited to people of lower socioeconomic status, which is reflected in the higher depression levels in this group (< 2,000 MYR). Through the PeKa B40 initiative, the government seeks to subsidise the management of non-communicable diseases for the bottom 40% of income earners. With regards to mental health, the initiative is currently limited to subsidising mental health screenings in private clinics to mitigate the limited workforce in the government hospitals. The expansion of this initiative, which is in the works, should include mental health treatments following screening. Remunerations for government mental health practitioners should be revised to recruit and retain well-qualified practitioners. These suggestions are justified given the substantial economic cost of mental illnesses (approximately 14.46 billion MYR) in Malaysia (Chua, 2020).

Assessing the mental health impact of the COVID-19 pandemic was difficult given the scarce pre-pandemic data. In light of this, mental health data should be streamlined and published for proper monitoring, evaluation, and analysis. Currently, different measures, variables, and exclusion criteria are used across the years (Institute for Public Health, 2020), resulting in fragmented data and futile trend analyses.

As discussed in the Introduction, another pressing mental health policy is the decriminalisation of suicide—which has led to decreased suicide rates in Malaysia's neighbouring country, Singapore (Chua & Rao, 2021). Decriminalisation would not only improve help-seeking behaviour (Chong et al., 2013), but allow accurate data collection. Overall, greater transparency, with regards to mental health action plans and data, would allow proper feedback and monitoring.

3.5.2 Scope and limitations

The generalisability of the results is subject to certain limitations. This study made use of non-probability sampling which can lead to a bias in the results. Individuals with existing mental health conditions or aged 75 and older are not frequent internet users and therefore, the internet-based sample used might be an underrepresentation of those who are most in need (Office for National Statistics, 2019; Pierce et al., 2020a). This is evident by the high number of respondents who have tertiary education. Moreover, females were overrepresented in the study. Furthermore, the survey was conducted a week after the MCO was replaced with CMCO, but participants were asked to answer based on their experience in the past 2 weeks. Therefore, the results contain participants' experiences during both CMCO and MCO. Notwithstanding these limitations, the survey was conducted in both English as Bahasa Malaysia to include a more diverse and larger sample, thus increasing statistical power.

Practical suggestions

Despite the high reliance on internet-based communication during the pandemic, our findings suggest that individuals should limit their daily use of social media. Interventions that are affordable, culturally sensitive and easily accessible to mitigate logistical and financial barriers, should be designed and targeted toward these individuals with identified risk factors (e.g. history of mental health services, lower income and unemployment).

Acknowledgement

This work was supported by the Research Management Center at HELP University via the Internal Research Grant Scheme (No. 20-04-015).

Note

1. Residents who reside in Malaysia with 97.10% being Malaysians.

References

Chan, C. M. H., Ng, S. L., In, S., Wee, L. H., & Siau, C. S. (2021). Predictors of psychological distress and mental health resource utilization among employees in Malaysia. *International Journal of Environmental Research and Public Health*, *18*(1), 314. DOI: 10.3390/ijerph18010314

Chong, S., Mohamad, M. S., & Er, A. C. (2013). The mental health development in Malaysia: History, current issue and future development. *Asian Social Science*, *9*(6), 1–8. DOI: 10.5539/ass.v9n6p1

Chua, S. N. (2020). The economic cost of mental disorders in Malaysia. *The Lancet Psychiatry*, *7*(4), e23. DOI: 10.1016/S2215-0366(20)30091-2

Chua, S. N., & Rao, M. V. (2021). Youth suicide in Malaysia. *Relate Mental Health Malaysia*. Retrieved from https://www.ideas.org.my/publications/reports/

Classen, T. J., & Dunn, R. A. (2012). The effect of job loss and unemployment duration on suicide risk in the United States: A new look using mass-layoffs and unemployment duration. *Health Economy*, *21*(3), 338–350. DOI: 10.1038/jid.2014.371

Dalgard, O. S. (1996). Community health profile as a tool for psychiatric prevention. In D. R. Trent & C. Reeds C. (Eds.), *Promotion of mental health*. United Kingdom: Ashgate Publishing.

Fiorillo, A., Sampogna, G., Giallonardo, V., Del Vecchio, V., Luciano, M., Albert, U., Carmassi, C., Carrà, G., Cirulli, F., Dell'Osso, B., Nanni, M. G., Pompili, M., Sani, G., Tortorella, A., & Volpe, U. (2020). Effects of the lockdown on the mental health of the general population during the COVID-19 pandemic in Italy: Results from the COMET collaborative network. *European Psychiatry*, *63*(1), e87.

Goldberg, D., & Williams, P. (1988). *A user's guide to the general health questionnaire*. Windsor, UK: NFER-Nelson.

Haque, A. (2005). Mental health concepts and program development in Malaysia. *Journal of Mental Health*, *14*(2), 183–195. DOI: 10.1080/09638230500059997

House of Senate (2020a). *3 December Debate*. https://www.parlimen.gov.my/files/jindex/pdf/JDR03122020.pdf

House of Senate (2020b). *23 December Debate*. https://www.parlimen.gov.my/files/hindex/pdf/DN-23122020.pdf

Institute for Public Health. (2015). *National health and morbidity survey 2015, Vol. II: Non-communicable diseases, risk factors & other health problems*. Kuala Lumpur: Institute for Public Health, National Institutes of Health, Ministry of Health Malaysia.

Institute for Public Health. (2020). National Health and Morbidity Survey 2019: Vol. I: NCDs – Non-Communicable Diseases: Risk Factors and other Health Problems. National Institutes of Health, Ministry of Health Malaysia.

Kader Maideen, S. F., Mohd Sidik, S., Rampal, L., & Mukhtar, F. (2015). Prevalence, associated factors and predictors of anxiety: A community survey in Selangor, Malaysia. *BMC Psychiatry*, *15*, 262. DOI: 10.1186/s12888-015-0648-x

Keles, B., McCrae, N., & Grealish, A. (2020). A systematic review: The influence of social media on depression, anxiety and psychological distress in adolescents, *International Journal of Adolescence and Youth*, *25* (1), 79–93. DOI: 10.1080/02673843.2019.1590851

Kocalevent, R. D., Berg, L., Beutel, M. E., Hinz, A., Zenger, M., Härter, M., Nater, U., & Brähler, E. (2018). Social support in the general population: Standardization of the Oslo social support scale (OSSS-3). *BMC Psychology*, *6*(1), 4–11. DOI: 10.1186/s40359-018-0249-9

Lim, S. L. (2018). Bridging Barriers: A Report on Improving Access to Mental Healthcare in Malaysia. Retrieved from https://penanginstitute.org/wp-content/uploads/jml/files/research_papers/PenangInstituteinKL_Bridging%20Barriers%20Report_LimSuLin_2ndJanuary2018_final.pdf

Lovibond, S. H., & Lovibond, P. F. (1995). *Manual for the Depression Anxiety Stress Scales* (2nd ed.). Sydney: Psychology Foundation of Australia.

Lundin, A., Åhs, J., Åsbring, N., Kosidou, K., Dal, H., Tinghög, P., Saboonchi, F., & Dalman, C. (2017). Discriminant validity of the 12-item version of the general health questionnaire in a Swedish case-control study. *Nordic Journal of Psychiatry*, *71*, 171–179. DOI: 10.1080/08039488.2016.1246608

Ministry of Health (MOH). (2021). Ministry of Health: Official Portal. Retrieved from https://www.moh.gov.my/

Munawar, K., Mukhtar, F., Choudhry, F. R., & Ng, A. L. O. (2021). Mental health literacy: A systematic review of knowledge and beliefs about mental disorders in Malaysia. *Asia Pac Psychiatry*, *May 8*, e12475. DOI: 10.1111/appy.12475

News Straits Times. (2020, March 31). Befrienders KL sees more calls during MCO. *News Straits Times*. Retrieved from https://www.nst.com.my/news/nation/2020/03/580036/befrienders-kl-sees-more-calls-during-mco

Office for National Statistics. (2019). Office for National Statistics. Internet users. Retrieved from https://www.ons.gov.uk/businessindustryandtrade/itandinternetindustry/bulletins/internetusers/2019

Pierce, M., Hope, H., Ford, T., Hatch, S., Hotopf, M., John, A., Kontopantelis, E., Webb, R., Wessely, S., McManus, S., & Abel, K. M. (2020b). Mental health before and during the COVID-19 pandemic: A longitudinal probability sample survey of the UK population. *The Lancet Psychiatry*, *7*(10), 883–892. DOI: 10.1016/S2215-0366(20)30308-4

Pierce, M., McManus, S., Jessop, C., John, A., Hotopf, M., Ford, T., Hatch, S., Wessely, S., & Abel, K. M. (2020a). Says who? The significance of sampling in mental health surveys during COVID-19. *The Lancet Psychiatry*, *7*(7), 567–568. DOI: 10.1016/S2215-0366(20)30237-6

Relate Mental Health Malaysia. (2020). Workplace mental health: The business costs. Kuala Lumpur.

Rens, E., Smith, P., Nicaise, P., Lorant, V., & Van den Broeck, K. (2021). Mental distress and its contributing factors among young people during the first wave of COVID-19: A Belgian survey study. *Frontiers in Psychiatry, 12*(January). DOI: 10.3389/fpsyt.2021.575553

Shah, A. U. M., Safri, S. N. A., Thevadas, R., Noordin, N. K., Rahman, A. A., Sekawi, Z., Ideris, A., & Sultan, M. T. H. (2020). COVID-19 outbreak in Malaysia: Actions taken by the Malaysian government. *International Journal of Infectious Diseases, 97*, 108–116. DOI: 10.1016/j.ijid.2020.05.093

Swader, C. S. (2019). Loneliness in Europe: Personal and societal individualism-collectivism and their connection to social isolation. *Social Forces, 97*(3), 1307–1336. DOI: 10.1093/sf/soy088

Vassall, A., Sweeney, S., Barasa, E., Prinja, S., Keogh-Brown, M. R., Tarp Jensen, H., Smith, R., Baltussen, R., Eggo, R. M., & Jit, M. (2020). Integrating economic and health evidence to inform covid-19 policy in low-and middle-income countries. *Wellcome Open Research, 5*, 272. DOI: 10.12688/wellcomeopenres.16380.1

Wang, C., Tee, M., Roy, A. E., Fardin, M. A., Srichokchatchawan, W., Habib, H. A., Tran, B. X., Hussain, S., Hoang, M. T., Le, X. T., Ma, W., Pham, H. Q., Shirazi, M., Taneepanichskul, N., Tan, Y., Tee, C., Xu, L., Xu, Z., Vu, G. T., & Kuruchittham, V. (2021). The impact of COVID-19 pandemic on physical and mental health of Asians: A study of seven middle-income countries in Asia. *PloS One, 16*(2), e0246824. DOI: 10.1371/journal.pone.0246824

WHO. (2018). Managing epidemics. Retrieved from https://www.who.int/emergencies/diseases/managing-epidemics-interactive.pdf

Xiong, J., Lipsitz, O., Nasri, F., Lui, L. M. W., Gill, H., & Phan, L. (2020). Impact of COVID-19 pandemic on mental health in the general population: A systematic review. *Journal of Affective Disorders Journal, 277*, 55–64.

Yap, A. E., Daojuin, D. L., Jingqi, H., Sim, I., Wong, J., & Firdaus, M. S. (2020). Improving accessibility and availability of mental health services in Malaysia. Malaysianmedics.Org (June).

Zhou, L. K., Tang, S., & Arulthevan, N. Y. (2021). Post COVID-19 recovery: Building SME resilience. *Policy Ideas* (January).

4 Women's emotional health and support in a time of crisis

Vimala Balakrishnan, Kee Seong Ng, &
Azmawaty Mohamad Nor

4.1 Introduction

Malaysia is currently experiencing an upsurge of COVID-19 cases, with more than 550,000 recorded as of May 27, 2021 (Worldometer, 2021). The Phase 1 of a nationwide lockdown was imposed on March 18, 2020, and further extended to several states such as Selangor and Kuala Lumpur till January 14, 2021. It was further extended to Phase 2 (up to June 9, 2020) and the local media has highlighted the increase in emotional distress particularly among women. The Women, Family and Community Development Ministry reported an increase of 57% of distress-related calls from women during the lockdown whereas the Women's Aid Organization (WAO) reported a 150% increase in hotline calls and an 80% increase in WhatsApp messages distress channel compared to 2019 (Sukumaran, 2020). For example, distress calls received from women include juggling between work and life, lack of support received from family members and employers, domestic abuse and violence cases and lack of income; just to name a few. An elevated distress among women were observed globally as well, for example, violence against Tunisian women were found to have increased from 4% to 14.8% during the COVID-19 lockdown, with the majority having experienced extreme severe depression, stress and anxiety levels (Sediri et al., 2020).

Studies particularly targeting women are scarce both locally and globally. In fact, a search of the literature revealed a vast majority of COVID-19 and emotional health-related studies focused more on the prevalence rates among general population, health practitioners and university students, with very few targeting women (Lahav, 2020; Sediri et al., 2020; Wang et al., 2020b). Local media reports on the negative consequences of COVID-19 and lockdown are in abundance, however, only two empirical studies examining the distress level of Malaysian university students were found (Kalok et al., 2020; Kamaludin et al., 2020). Further, none

DOI: 10.4324/9781003178576-6

of these studies focused on the emotional support system adopted by the affected population. Only the work of Kamaludin et al. (2020) examined students' coping strategies, with results indicating students who are highly anxious tend to seek social support compared to others. A good support system plays an important role in mitigating the risks of emotional distress amongst women, therefore; this warrants an investigation (Harandi et al., 2017). Women are often regarded as kin-keepers of a family; hence, they are overwhelmed in having to manage their households and children, working from home, etc. For example, females with a higher number of children with lack of social support were found to be positively associated with a higher level of emotional distress during COVID-19 isolation (Le et al., 2020). The impact of the lockdown on women's emotional state needs to be examined and addressed to help them cope psychologically not only during the lockdown period but post-lockdown as well.

Therefore, in order to address these gaps and extend the literature, the present study aims to determine the prevalence rate of emotional distress among Malaysian women (aged more than 25), the socio-demographic correlates and the emotional support systems adopted during the crisis. We specifically define emotional distress during the nationwide lockdown as a form of negative effect to an individual's emotional health due to stress and depression (further details in the Methodology section). A search of the literature revealed several studies that have particularly focused on specific mental or emotional health aspects, including stress, anxiety, depression etc. For instance, Sriharan et al. (2020) investigated the stress and depression symptoms among women and found that these two variables are significantly associated with mental health issues. Yan et al. (2021) specifically focused on stress and found women to more likely experience stress during the Covid-19 pandemic than men, whereas Lin et al. (2020) found 34.7% of their college student participants to have experienced depression with those with higher masculinity traits to less likely experience depression.

Others found students who were affected by prolonged school closure to experience severe psychological stress, which may increase the likelihood of depression. Additionally, studies suggest that women who experience domestic violence and abuse especially during the lockdown have a higher risk of developing depressive symptoms (Mapayi et al., 2013). Therefore, with the emotional distress spike being reported and the on-going pandemic and lockdowns, the study is deemed timely. Further, it is believed that the identification of the socio-demographic correlates and emotional support systems will provide useful insights to the relevant authorities including mental health practitioners, counsellors, etc. so that vulnerable women or cohorts can be identified, and immediate and appropriate intervention and coping strategies could be devised to help the women cope better.

4.1.1 Research questions

The study is guided by the following research questions (RQs):

RQ1 – What is the prevalence rate of emotional distress among Malaysian women during the nationwide lockdown?

RQ2 – Which socio-demographic factors predict emotional distress in women?

RQ3 – What emotional support system(s) are adopted by women?

RQ4 – Which socio-demographic factors predict the need for emotional support?

4.2 Literature review

Women are generally deemed to be more susceptible to emotional distress as they usually have to shoulder key responsibilities at home including as the main caregiver, kin-keeper, juggling work and children etc., and often with unequal burden of parenting and household chore management compared to their male counterparts. Studies focusing on the women and their emotional health or well-being are in paucity, except for a few who reported elevated distress levels among their women participants. For example, women with COVID-19 symptoms and poor perceived health were found to show higher levels of depression and anxiety in China (Wang et al., 2020a) whilst younger females living alone and not in a relationship experienced more distress in Israel (Lahav, 2020). In Tunisia, women with a history of mental illness and who were abused during COVID-19 lockdown exhibited extremely severe symptoms of depression (57%) and stress (53.1%) (Sediri et al., 2020). The authors also found age to be significantly and negatively correlated with depression, stress and anxiety, a finding that was echoed in a study involving 3,063 social media users in China (Hou et al., 2020). The authors found the severity of depression to be negatively associated with age, and positively associated with being unemployed. On the other hand, females were found to be more stressed and anxious than males, specifically those who spent more than an hour on information related to COVID-19.

Malaysian-based studies revealed female students below 25 years and living alone to have experienced a high level of anxiety (Kamaludin et al., 2020). The authors also explored the students' coping strategies with findings indicating individuals with a high level of anxiety tend to seek more social support compared to others who accept the situation (i.e. maladaptive behaviour). Another

Malaysian study among 772 clinical undergraduates found female students displayed higher scores for depression, anxiety and stress compared to males (Kalok et al., 2020). Appropriate emotional support is important in alleviating anxiety and stress and promoting greater mental well-being amongst students during the nationwide quarantine. In another study conducted on the Malaysian public 2 months after the onset of the pandemic, findings indicated that there were increased depressive, anxiety and stress symptoms. Students, women and people in poor financial situation were found to be emotionally distressed (Wong et al., 2021). The social demographic that was observed in the studies conducted during the pandemic include age, education, marital status, total household income, household size and living condition (Kalok et al., 2020; Kamaludin et al., 2020; Wong, et al., 2021).

Further, studies have been carried out on the association of social support with stress and coping mechanisms during the outbreak of influenza (Pressman et al., 2005), Ebola (Mohammed et al., 2015) as well as COVID-19 (Xiao et al., 2020) with results indicating a good social support system greatly contributes to physical and emotional health. Although the majority of the studies cite social ties such as family, friends and peers to be the main source of support, it is also important to explore a more formal support (e.g. mental health experts or community organisations) (Li et al., 2021). This is especially true during crises such as a pandemic as individuals face a multitude of stressful events due to the pandemic and its related consequences (e.g. prolonged lockdowns, isolations, etc.). Interestingly, individuals are also known to handle the crisis on their own by practicing or adapting various measures. For instance, Martin et al. (2021) found a significant increase in the use of music as a form of emotional self-regulation during isolation among Spaniards aged 51 years and above. Similarly, social work students were found to have adopted several emotional coping strategies, mainly self-sufficient, avoidant and socially supported mechanisms (Apgar & Cadmus, 2021).

4.3 Methodology

This study is part of a larger study that aims to identify the underlying motives predicting emotional distress among Malaysian women due to the COVID-19 lockdown, therefore only sections relevant to this study are presented.

4.3.1 Instrument and procedure

A self-reporting survey adapted from the Depression, Anxiety and Stress Scale (DASS)-21 and previous literature on support systems was developed in English, and further translated into the local language, Bahasa

Malaysia. Both versions were piloted, and minor amendments were made prior to the final survey distribution.

Ethical approval was sought from the Universiti Malaya Research Ethics Committee (UMREC). The target respondents were recruited based on three criteria, namely, gender (women), age (25 and above) and nationality (Malaysian). The survey questionnaire was hosted using Google Form and the link was widely distributed through Facebook and WhatsApp (i.e. mobile messaging app). The data collection was administered from June 2 to June 9, 2020, resulting in 1,793 responses. Using $Z = 1.96$; population = 300,000; error estimates at 5% and confidence level at 95%, the sample size was established at 384 (Qualtrics, 2020). As we managed to gather a high number of valid responses, the data collection exercise was halted in a week. No personal details that can be used to identify the women were collected, hence anonymity was ensured.

4.3.2 Measures

There were four sections in the survey, as follows:

> Section A solicited the respondents' demographic profiles including age, marital status, total household income, household size and living condition, among others.
>
> Section B contained 14 statements from DASS-21 specifically focusing on the depressive and stress symptoms (Lovibond & Lovibond, 1995). These were measured using a scale ranging from 0 (not applicable) to 3 (applied to me very much). The sum scores were accumulated on the items per subscale and multiplied by a factor of 2, resulting in scores ranging between 0 and 42 for each subscale. The scores and categories for each of the sub-scale are as follows:
> Depression: Normal (0–9), mild (10–12), moderate (13–20), severe (21–27) and extremely severe (28–42), and
> Stress: Normal (0–10), mild (11–18), moderate (19–26), severe (27–34) and extremely severe (35–42)

The Bahasa Malaysia version for DASS-21 was adopted from Musa et al. (2007). The sub-scales were found to be reliable as per their respective Cronbach alpha scores, that is, $\alpha_{depressive} = 0.870$ and $\alpha_{stress} = 0.866$. The present study re-coded the outcome of these two sub-scales into emotional distress (binary variable). In other words, respondents who were identified as Normal in the depressive and stress sub-scales were labeled as No, and the rest were labeled as Yes for emotional distress (i.e. as long as one symptom is exhibited regardless of its severity level). The method adopted in re-coding the outcome of the depression and stress levels into a single factor known as emotional distress had been adopted in similar studies. For example, Kalok et al. (2020) who investigated psychological impacts of lockdown among clinical undergraduates re-coded depression, anxiety and stress into a factor known as psychological distress. The authors defined a respondent who demonstrated symptoms of depression, anxiety, or stress from the calculated scores to be deemed as experiencing psychological distress. A similar re-coding of the depression and stress scores was also administered in our previous work (Balakrishnan et al., 2021).

Section C measured the underlying motives for the emotional distress such as financial issues, marital issues and personal issues. This section is not elaborated further as it is not part of the present study. Further details of this section and the related results are available in Balakrishnan et al. (2021).

Section D comprised items adapted from previous studies that showed individuals often depend on social ties such as family, friends (Pressman et al., 2005; Mohammed et al., 2015; Xiao et al., 2020) and also formal support (Li et al., 2021) to cope psychologically. Further, self-management or being self-sufficient has been reported as one of the coping mechanisms (Apgar & Cadmus, 2021; Martin et al., 2021). Specifically, there were five items in this section (see Table 4.3), with an alpha score of $\alpha = 0.701$, all measured using the same scale used in Section C. To be precise, a Likert scale was used to assess all the items in C and D (0 – Not relevant; 1 – Strongly disagree; 4 – Strongly agree). Further, the neutral point was omitted to eliminate the possibility that respondents will misuse the midpoint, which is a common issue in self-reporting questionnaires as shown by numerous studies comparing the five-point and four-point Likert scales (Chyung et al., 2017; Kulas & Stachowski, 2009). As the items were intended to examine the support system adopted by the women under-study to manage their emotional health, this particular construct is referred to as emotional support in this study.

4.3.3 Data analysis

The Statistical Package for Social Sciences (SPSS) 26 was used to analyse the collected data. Mean, frequencies and percentages were used to describe the data whereas binary logistic regressions were administered to identify the emotional distress predictors (i.e. emotional distress as a binary variable and as the dependent variable). On the other hand, linear regressions were administered to determine the socio-demographic predictors for emotional support (i.e. as an interval variable, and as the dependent variable). All the significance tests were set at $p < 0.05$.

4.4 Findings

4.4.1 Women respondents

Table 4.1 provides the demographic details of the women in our study. A majority of them were between 31 and 60 years old (78.6%) and working from home (61.6%). Most of the respondents were Malays, followed by Chinese and Indians, in line with the ethnicity distribution in the country. It can also be observed that a majority of the women had a tertiary education and above (92.8%), and only less than 1% with a primary education. Married women make up most of the sample (70.5%), and majority were staying with their families (85.9%). Approximately, 93% of the women reported a household size between 2 and 9, with a majority household monthly income between 3,001 and 10,000 MYR (750–2500 USD) (53.7%).

Table 4.1 Demographics of the women respondents

Variables	Categories	Frequency	%	Variables	Categories	Frequency	%
Age	24–30	338	18.9	Marital status	Married	1264	70.5
	31–40	645	36.0		Single with kids	85	4.7
	41–60	764	42.6		Single without kids	444	24.8
	61 and above	46	2.6	Living condition	Alone	156	8.7
Ethnicity	Malay	1368	76.3		Co-sharing	97	5.4
	Chinese	186	10.4		Family	1540	85.9
	Indian	174	9.7	Household size	1	91	5.1
	Others	65	3.6		2–4	859	47.9
Status	Student	145	8.1		5–9	808	45.1
	Work from home	1105	61.6		More than 10	35	2.0
	Essential/ Front liners	274	15.3	Total household monthly income (MYR)	Less than 3K	319	17.8
	Unemployed/ homemaker/ retired	224	12.5		3001–10000	963	53.7
	Loss of Job	25	1.4		10001–25000	402	22.4
	Others	20	1.1		More than 25K	109	6.1
Education	Primary	7	0.4				
	Secondary	123	6.9				
	Tertiary	815	45.5				
	Postgraduate	848	47.3				

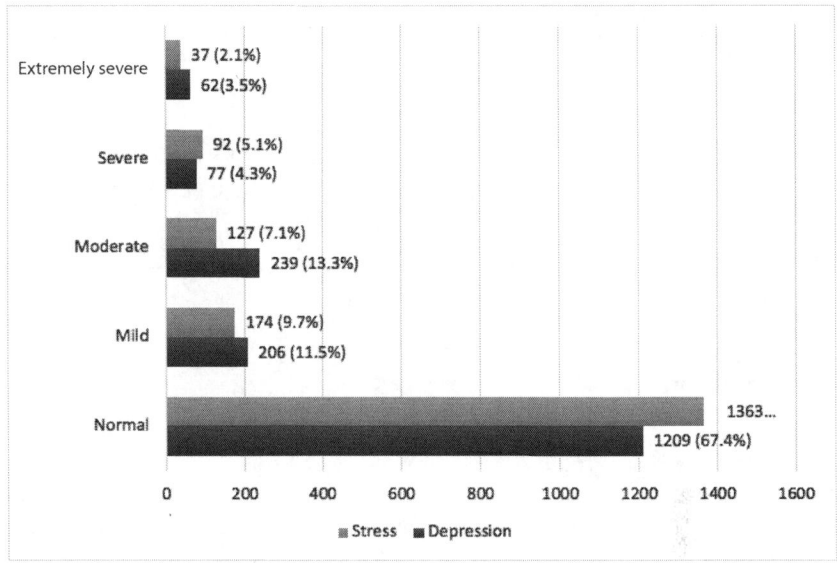

Figure 4.1 Depression and stress prevalence rates based on their severity levels.

4.4.2 Emotional distress prevalence rate

To answer our first research question, frequencies and percentages for the sub-scales are provided in Figure 4.1. The majority of the women were in the normal category, however, of those who exhibit distress symptoms, more women were found to be depressed than stressed (except for the severe category). The majority were found to fall between mild and moderate levels of depression (24.8%) and stress (16.8%), whilst the remaining exhibited a higher level of depression (7.8%; $N = 139$) and stress (7.2%; $N = 129$) symptoms. In terms of emotional distress categorisation, approximately 37% ($N = 669$) of the women experienced emotional distress to a certain extent whilst the remaining did not exhibit any (63%; $N = 1124$). The prevalence rates were determined as per the re-coding described in Methodology.

4.4.3 Emotional distress predictors

Table 4.2 answers our RQ2, with results indicating age ($p < 0.001$) and total household income ($p = 0.015$) to significantly predict emotional distress among the women, whereas the rest of the socio-demographics were found to be insignificant. The negative relationships further indicate that as age and total monthly household income increase, emotional distress decreases.

Table 4.2 Binary logistic regressions for emotional distress

Factors	ß	Wald	P - value
Age	−0.486	46.04	0.000[a]
Total household income (monthly)	−0.181	5.89	0.015[a]
Marital Status	0.051	0.549	0.459
Living condition	−0.008	0.007	0.931
Household size	−0.096	1.137	0.286
Education level	0.052	0.398	0.528

[a] Significant at $\alpha < 0.05$

4.4.4 Emotional distress and support

In order to answer the third research question, descriptive statistics were administered (see Table 4.3). The majority of the women in this study were found to self-manage ($M = 3.31$; $N = 626$) suggesting a cohort that is resilient. The second popular support system among the women were family members ($M = 3.04$; $N = 520$). Social media/online platforms and professionals emerged to be the least favoured support system among the women as indicated by the low mean values (all below 3.00) and frequencies.

A further execution of the binary logistic regression revealed emotional support does not significantly predict emotional distress among the women ($p = 0.291$).

Table 4.3 Descriptive statistics for emotional support

Emotional support items	Mean (Standard deviation)	N (%)
I self-manage	3.31 (0.583)	626 (76.6)
I turn to my family members for emotional support	3.04 (0.725)	520 (29.0)
I turn to my friends for emotional support	2.91 (0.683)	514 (28.7)
I turn to social media/online for emotional support	2.20 (0.832)	284 (42.5)
I turn to professionals (counsellors, NGO, etc.) for emotional support	2.16 (0.791)	208 (31.1)

Note: Total does not tally to 1,793 as multiple selections were allowed; The *N* and % in the last column were determined using crosstab tabulations (i.e. aggregation of agree and strongly agree for each item).

Table 4.4 Linear regression for emotional support

Factors	ß	t-value	p-value
Age	−0.013	−0.500	0.617
Total household income (monthly)	−0.086	−2.810	0.005[a]
Marital status	−0.051	−0.831	0.190
Living condition	−0.008	−0.440	0.731
Household size	−0.006	−0.407	0.770
Education level	−0.140	−3.670	0.001[a]

[a] Significant at $\alpha < 0.05$.

4.4.5 Socio-demographic factors and emotional support

As for RQ4, linear regressions revealed education level (ß $= -0.140$; $t = -3.67$; $p < 0.001$) and total monthly household income (ß $= -0.086$; $t = -2.81$; $p = 0.005$) to significantly predict emotional support, as shown in Table 4.4. The negative coefficients indicate that women with lower education and income levels emphasize more on emotional support compared to the rest of the women.

4.5 Conclusion

The COVID-19 pandemic has impacted the lives of many throughout the world, and Malaysia is not exempted. Resulting lockdowns due to the pandemic caused severe disruptions to the social norms, with women being more susceptible to emotional distress. The present study was therefore conducted to examine the prevalence of emotional distress among Malaysian women during COVID-19 lockdown, a period that observed increased mental health issues both globally and locally. The study specifically examined the emotional support system received/adopted by the women.

4.5.1 Emotional distress prevalence among the women

Key findings indicate Malaysian women to have somewhat experienced emotional distress (i.e. 37%), slightly lower than those reported by Kalok et al. (2020), who found 52.8% of their clinical undergraduates in Malaysia to have experienced distress due to COVID-19 lockdown, the latter of which also utilised DASS-21 scale. Similarly, the depression and stress levels were found to be lower than those reported in Kalok et al. (2020) (i.e. 24% vs 32.6%; 27.5% vs 36% for depression and stress, respectively). The two different samples targeted by the studies clearly indicate the varying levels of distress among Malaysians, with the women having experienced a lower level of emotional distress compared to university students. Interestingly, the former cohort shoulders a heavier responsibility including (single) parenting, juggling work and children, working from home, financial concerns and uncertainties compared to students who were mostly worried about online learning, future academic and career prospects.

On the other hand, the distress rates among our women were exceedingly lower than those experienced by Tunisian women (Sediri et al., 2020). In fact, the authors reported a very high (82.3%) and (82%) rates for depression and stress levels (Sediri et al., 2020), probably because their sample comprised more women who have been abused prior to the lockdown; in fact, their findings also indicate the violence rate to have increased significantly during the COVID-19 lockdown (14.8%).

4.5.2 Socio-demographic factors

Our results also indicate age and total household income to predict women's emotional distress, with younger women and those with lower-income levels having experienced a higher level of distress, concurring with several studies (Lahav, 2020; Sediri et al., 2020). The higher emotional distress among younger women could be associated with their increased online activities, a pattern that has been observed in several studies whereby a spike in social media use seeking news and information related to COVID-19 have been reported (Hou et al., 2021; Hou et al., 2020). In fact, Hou et al. (2020) reported their female social media users who spent more than an hour daily on COVID-19 related information to be more stressed and anxious.

Younger women are also considered to be less successful in maintaining a positive attitude in adapting to the new social norms, a notion that is supported by the Socio-emotional Selectivity Theory (SST), an emotional regulation theory of aging whereby humans prioritize their goals based on the current stages of life in maximising their life satisfaction (Carstensen, 2006). Older age is usually related to a shorter lifetime; thus, they tend to prioritise goals related to optimizing their affective well-being. This suggests that they may pay more attention to positive information and less on negative information to optimize their affective well-being, hence are less susceptible to emotional distress compared to the younger women.

The study also found women with lower education and income levels emphasised more on emotional support. Women sharing similar characteristics have been shown to experience more severe depressive symptoms in several studies (Sediri et al., 2020; Papageorge et al., 2020). Similarly, women with higher education may already have a good support system or are capable of managing the crisis independently; hence, they are not overly concerned about support systems unlike those with lower education. A higher household income may be associated with higher levels of self-protective behaviours resulting in a low level of emotional distress (Papageorge et al., 2020). This could suggest that if the low household income people do not have an avenue to increase their earning power, this could lead to more significant emotional distress and bad health conditions. The support from the government of Malaysia in providing more home-based job opportunities may help improve the emotional well-being of the affected women by reducing their distress level and ensuring a steady flow of income to maintain their lifestyle.

Additionally, monetary assistance from the government and allowing money to be withdrawn from the Employee Provident Fund were among the ways to mitigate the financial crisis faced by affected households. Further financial support was given in the form of subsidised utility bills. To top it off, Talian Kasih platform provides an avenue for the women to externalise their feelings and seek help from counsellors.

Interestingly, other factors such as marital status, living condition and household size did not significantly predict emotional support among the women in this study. The lockdown has witnessed a slowdown in activities throughout the nation, with most family members being together under one roof. This could result in family members and the communities having more time to provide support to each other.

4.5.3 Emotional distress and support systems

The women were also found to be quite resilient considering emotional support was found not to predict their emotional distress, and the fact that they mostly face and handle their problems on their own and with the support of their family members. This can be attributed to the fact that the majority of the women in this study are well-educated (i.e. more than 90% with at least a university degree) and employed, thus possessing the ability and skill to adjust and contain the bad or negative mood caused by the pandemic.

The emergence of family members as the second most popular emotional support among the women is also in accordance with Kalok et al. (2020) who demonstrated that students with a good family support experienced lower distress levels and higher mental well-being than those without. Family support system is somewhat unsurprising considering the importance Asians place on family relationships, where it is considered natural for family members to help each other, give priority and preference to one another at the expense of non-family members (Yaacob, 2005). The majority of the women in this study are married and living with their family (i.e. husband and children), hence the finding may suggest that these women turn to their spouses for emotional support.

Social media/online platforms and professionals emerged to be the least favoured emotional support system. This perhaps can be attributed to the Asian culture as well where there is a tendency to feel shy or uncomfortable in sharing personal or intimate family issues with an outsider (Kramer et al., 2002). In fact, Malaysian women may take the proverbial adage *"don't wash your dirty linen in public"* a tad seriously albeit the education and urbanization. The women may also see this as a sign of weakness as they had to resort to professionals instead of being able to handle their crisis privately, or within a circle of family members and close friends.

In general, our findings revealed emotional distress to be prevalent among Malaysian women, and specific socio-demographics that require further assistance (i.e. women with lower education and income levels). These women are identified as the most vulnerable cohort; hence relevant authorities should emphasise specific intervention strategies. For example, special initiatives can be introduced in the form of home-based businesses (both online and offline) to help women improve their income levels. Additionally, relevant business-related training can be introduced to help these women to better equip themselves with the necessary knowledge and skill. Finally, specific platforms can be developed and introduced to support individuals who were psychologically affected due to the pandemic and lockdowns. The intervention and coping strategies are of paramount importance considering that the country is currently experiencing an upsurge of COVID-19 cases, which have resulted in partial lockdowns in several states.

4.5.4 Scope and limitations

This study, however, has several limitations. Firstly, the data were primarily collected through an online medium; therefore, women from a disadvantaged background (e.g. rural areas, poor Internet locations, etc.) were excluded. The findings of the study are, therefore, to be interpreted with caution. The use of online data collection also resulted in another limitation, that is, location. A vast majority of the women were from urban areas;

therefore, a location-based analysis was not possible (e.g. comparison between East and West Malaysia). Future studies could explore this avenue as well.

Practical suggestions

Emphasis on specific intervention strategies is recommended, for example, special initiatives can be introduced in the form of home-based businesses (online and offline) to help women improve their income levels, and relevant business-related training can be introduced to help these women to better equip themselves with the necessary knowledge and skill. Finally, specific platforms can be developed to support individuals psychologically affected due to the pandemic and lockdowns.

Acknowledgement

This work was supported by the Universiti Malaya Special COVID-19 Grant [CSRG002-2020SS].

References

Apgar, D., & Cadmus, T. (2021). Using mixed methods to assess the coping and self-regulation skills of undergraduate social work students impacted by COVID-19. *Clinical Social Work Journal*. DOI: 10.1007/s10615-021-00790-3

Balakrishnan, V., Nor, A. M., & Zainal, N. Z. (2021). COVID-19 nationwide lockdown and its emotional stressors among Malaysian women, *Asia Pacific Journal of Social Work and Development*. DOI: 10.1080/02185385.2021.1886976

Carstensen, L. L. (2006). The influence of a sense of time on human development. *Science, 312*, 1913–1915.

Chyung, S. Y. Y., Roberts, K., Swanson, I., & Hankinson, A. (2017). Evidence-based survey design: The use of a midpoint on the Likert scale, *Performance Improvement, 56*, 15–23.

Harandi, T. F., Taghinasab, M. M., & Nayeri, T. D. (2017). The correlation of social support with mental health: A meta-analysis. *Electron Physician, 9*(9), 5212–5222.

Hou, F., Bi, F., Jiao, R., Luo, D., & Song, K. (2020). Gender differences of depression and anxiety among social media users during the COVID-19 outbreak in China: A cross-sectional study, *BMC Public Health, 20*. DOI: 10.1186/s12889-020-09738-7

Hou, K., Hou, T., & Cai, L. (2021). Public attention about COVID-19 on social media: An investigation based on data mining and text analysis. *Personality and Individual Differences, 175*, 110701

Kalok, A., Sharip, S., Hafizz, A. M. A., Zainuddin, Z. M., & Shafiee, M. N. (2020). The psychological impact of movement restriction during the COVID-19 outbreak on clinical undergraduates: A cross-sectional study. *International Journal of Environmental Research and Public Health, 17*(22), 8522.

Kamaludin, K., Chinna, K., Sundarasen, S., Khoshaim, H. B., Nurunnabi, M., Baloch, G. M., Sukayt, A., & Hossain, S. F. A. (2020). Coping with COVID-19 and movement control order (MCO): Experiences of university students in Malaysia. *Heliyon, 6*(11), e05339.

Kramer, E. J., Kwong, K., Lee, E., & Chung, H. (2020). Cultural factors influencing the mental health of Asian americans. *Western Journal of Medicine, 176*(4), 227–231.

Kulas, J. T., & Stachowski, A. A. (2009). Middle category endorsement in odd-numbered likert response scales: Associated item characteristics, cognitive demands, and preferred meanings. *Journal of Research in Personality, 43*(3), 489–493.

Lahav, Y. (2020). Psychological distress related to COVID-19 – The contribution of continuous traumatic stress. *Journal of Affective Disorder, 1*(277), 129–137.

Le, X. T. T., Dang, A. K., Toweh, J., Nguyen, Q. N., Le, H. T., Do, T. T. T., Phan, H. B. T., Nguyen, T. T., Pham, Q. T., Ta, N. K. T., Nguyen, Q. T., Nguyen, A. N., Duong, Q. V., Hoang, M. T., Pham, H. Q., Vu, L. G., Tran, B. T., Latkin, C. A., Ho, C. S. H., & Ho, R. C. M. (2020). Evaluating the psychological impacts related to COVID-19 of Vietnamese people under the first nationwide partial lockdown in Vietnam. *Frontiers in Psychiatry, 11.* DOI: 10.3389/fpsyt.2020.00824

Li, F., Luo, S., Mu, W., Li, Y., Ye, L., Zheng, X., Xu, B., Ding, Y., Ling, P., Zhou, M., & Chen, X. (2021). Effects of sources of social support and resilience on the mental health of different age groups during the COVID-19 pandemic. *BMC Psychiatry, 21*(16). DOI: 10.1186/s12888-020-03012-1

Lin, J., Guo, T., Becker, B., Yu, Q., Chen, S. T., Brendon, S., Hossain, M. M., Cunha, P. M., Soares, F. C., Veroneses, N., Yu, J. J., Grabovac, I., Smith, L., Yeung, A., Zhou, L., & Li, H. (2020). Depression is associated with moderate-intensity physical activity among college students during the COVID-19 pandemic: Differs by activity level, gender and gender role, *Psychology Research and Behavior Management, 13*, 1123–1134

Lovibond, P. F., & Lovibond, S. H. (1995). The structure of negative emotional states: Comparison of the depression anxiety stress scales (DASS) with the beck depression and anxiety inventories. *Behaviour Research and Therapy, 33*(3), 335–343.

Mapayi, B., Makanjuola, R. O. A., Mosaku, S. K., Adewuya, O. A., Afolabi, O., Aloba, O. O., & Akinsulore, A. (2013). Impact of intimate partner violence on anxiety and depression amongst women in ile-ife, Nigeria. *Archives of Women's Mental Health, 16*(1), 11–18.

Martin, J. C., Ignacio, D. O., Gracia, N. M., & Martin, M. G. (2021). Music as a factor associated with emotional self-regulation: A study on its relationship to age during COVID-19 lockdown in Spain. *Heliyon, 7*(2), e06274.

Mohammed, A., Sheikh, T. L., Gidado, S., Poggensee, G., Nguku, P., & Olayinka, A. (2015). An evaluation of psychological distress and social support of survivors and contacts of Ebola virus disease infection and their relatives in Lagos, Nigeria: A cross sectional study. *BMC Public Health*, *15*(1), 1–8.

Musa, R., Fadzil, M.A., & Zain, Z. (2007) Translation, validation and psychometric properties of Bahasa Malaysia version of the depression anxiety and stress scales (DASS), *ASEAN Journal of Psychiatry*, *8*(2), 82–89.

Papageorge, N. W., Zahn, M. V., Belot, M., van den Broek-Altenburg, E., Choi, S., Jamison, J. C., & Tripodi, E. (2020). Socio-demographic factors associated with self-protecting behavior during the COVID-19 pandemic. Retrieved from https://www.nber.org/papers/w27378, Accessed November 15, 2020

Pressman, S. D., Cohen, S., Miller, G. E., Barkin, A., Rabin, B. S., & Treanor, J. J. (2005). Loneliness, social network size, and immune response to influenza vaccination in college freshmen. *Health Psychology*, *24*(3), 297.

Qualtrics (2020) Sample size calculator, Retrieved from https://www.qualtrics.com/blog/calculating-sample-size/, Accessed January 2021.

Sediri, S., Zgueb, Y., Ouanes, S., Ouali, U., Bourgou, S., Jomli, R., & Nacef, F. (2020). Women's mental health: Acute impact of COVID-19 pandemic on domestic violence. *Archives of Women's Mental Health*, 23(6), 1–8.

Sriharan, A., Ratnapalan, S., Tricco, A., Lupea, D., Ayala, A. P., Pang, H., & Lee, D. D. (2020). Occupational stress, burnout and depression in women in healthcare during COVID-19 pandemic: A rapid scoping review. *Frontiers in Global Women's Health*, *1*, 20.

Sukumaran, T. (2020) Malaysian women, children bear brunt of coronavirus lockdown, the Coronavirus pandemic. Retrieved from https://www.scmp.com/week-asia/health-environment/article/3113852/malaysian-women-children-bear-brunt-coronavirus (Accessed November 2020).

Wang, C., Pan, R., Wan, X., Tan, Y., Xu, L., Ho, C. S., & Ho, R. C. (2020a). Immediate psychological responses and associated factors during the initial stage of the 2019 coronavirus disease (COVID-19) epidemic among the general population in China. *International Journal of Environmental Research and Public Health*, *17*(5), 1729.

Wang, C., Pan, R., Wan, X., Tan, Y., Xu, L., McIntyre, R. S., Choo, F. N., Tran, B., Ho, R., Sharma, V. K., & Ho, C. (2020b) A longitudinal study on the mental health of general population during the COVID-19 epidemic in China. *Brain Behavior Immunity*, *87*, 40–48.

Wong, L. P., Alias, H., Md Fuzi, A. A., Omar, I. S., Mohamad Nor, A., Tan, M. P., Baranovich, D. L., Saari, C. Z., Hamzah, S. H., Cheong, K. W., Poon, C. H., Ramoo, V., Chong, C. C., Myint, K., Zainuddin, S., & Chung, I. (2021). Escalating progression of mental health disorders during the COVID-19 pandemic: Evidence from a nationwide survey. *PLoS ONE*, *16*(3), e0248916.

Worldometer (2021). https://www.worldometers.info/coronavirus/country/malaysia/

Xiao, H., Zhang, Y., Kong, D., Li, S., & Yang, N. (2020) The effects of social support on sleep quality of medical staff treating patients with coronavirus disease 2019 (COVID-19) in January and February 2020 in China. *Medical Science Monitor, 26*, e923549.

Yaacob, H. (2005) Unity in Malay family, *Journal Pengajian Melayu, 16*, 187–199.

Yan, S., Xu, R., Stratton, T. D., Kavcic, V., Luo, D., Hou, F., & Jiang, Y. (2021). Sex differences and psychological stress: Responses to the COVID-19 pandemic in China. *BMC Public Health, 21*(1), 1–8.

Section III

Developing resilience during the pandemic

5 Psychological impact and the use of religious coping among Malaysian Catholic older adults

D. Gerard Joseph Louis, Clarence Devadass, Pauline Pooi Yin Leong, Melissa Shamini Perry, & Yuen Beng Lee

5.1 Introduction

The COVID-19 pandemic has caused a global health, political, economic and social crisis which has impacted the lives of communities and people all over the world in almost every way possible. In Malaysia, to curb the spread of the pandemic, the government imposed several phases of lockdowns, also known as Movement Control Orders (MCOs), since March 18, 2020. Due to the MCO, all large gatherings and events were suspended and public places including schools and places of worship were closed.

The Catholic Church in Malaysia adopted a very proactive stand to curb the pandemic. The Archbishops and Bishops in affected states promulgated that all Masses (*Mass is the central church worship service that is integral to the Catholic faith*) and church activities be suspended and churches, chapels, archdiocesan, diocesan and parish offices be closed even before the MCO was implemented (Archdiocese of Kuala Lumpur Media and Communications Office (AKLMCO), 2020). During this period, the Archbishops and Bishops dispensed the Catholic faithful from fulfilling their Sunday obligation of assisting or attending Mass and invited them to follow the Masses streamed online (AKLMCO, 2020). Although the suspension of religious activities and fellowship in churches was done in compliance with government regulations and in the interest of public health and safety, it affected approximately 2.5 million Catholics, or 7% of the Malaysian population of 33 million people as their ability to fulfil their religious obligations in churches was curtailed.

A notable impact of this pandemic on society has been the amplification of the digital divide as more and more people turned to technology to fulfil

DOI: 10.4324/9781003178576-8

their various needs. For the Catholics in Malaysia, the closure of churches meant that Masses were streamed online to help meet the spiritual needs of the Catholic faithful. In order to access the online Masses, members of the community had to increase their digital literacy. This proved a challenge for older adults, i.e. those aged 60 years and above (as defined in the 2011 Malaysian National Policy for Older Persons by the Ministry of Women, Family and Community Development), who were less technologically savvy. This rapid shift in moving Masses and other religious activities to a virtual platform led to a concern regarding the ability of the Catholic older adults to participate in these online activities. As revealed in a report by the Malaysian Communications and Multimedia Commission (MCMC, 2018), only 6.5% of older adults in Malaysia had access to the Internet (MCMC, 2018). In addition to the lack of accessibility to digital technology and Internet especially in rural areas (MCMC, 2018), older adults typically have more difficulty adjusting to new technologies due to a lack of technical experience, health status, complexities of new technology, frustration and need for dependence on others (Roupa et al., 2010).

Therefore, in the absence of effective coping strategies to adapt to new technology, norms and ways of living, the psychological well-being of older adults can be adversely impacted. In recognition of this, a qualitative case study was conducted to investigate the psychological impact of the pandemic on the well-being of Catholic older adults in Malaysia in the absence of face-to-face communal engagement, worship and pastoral support in churches. This chapter will discuss the challenges faced by Catholic older adults due to the disruption of spiritual, pastoral and social engagement and inaccessibility to Sacraments (*religious-ritual celebrations that Catholics believe impart God's grace through the external use of signs, symbols and prayers. There are seven Sacraments in the Catholic faith*). The chapter will also discuss religious coping strategies employed by older adults in response to these disruptions and include practical suggestions for the development of mechanisms to support their needs in times of such crisis.

5.2 Literature review

According to the World Health Organization (WHO), over 20% of adults over the age of 60 suffer from mental and neurological disorders, with depression (5%) and anxiety disorders (3.8%) being among the common mental health issues faced by this category of adults (WHO, 2017).

The current COVID-19 pandemic adds to concerns regarding the mental health of this segment of the population due to the effects of the stay-at-home orders, social distancing and lack of social support provided to this group of adults. These stay-at-home and social-distancing orders limit the ability to engage in meeting with friends and family, attend religious services, walks in the park, or even access prescribed nutrition, exacerbating possible increases in mental health issues among the older adults (Mukhtar, 2020). For example, Koma et al. (2020), in analysing the data from the US Census Bureau's Household Pulse Survey conducted between March 2020 to August 2020, found that almost a quarter of adults from 65 years and older reported having anxiety and depression compared with a tenth of such adults in 2018.

5.2.1 Resilience among older adults

Despite the seeming vulnerability of the older population to the psychological effects of the pandemic, studies have also shown that compared to younger members of the population, they seem to show a surprisingly greater level of resilience. In a study examining the level of resilience on COVID-19 Phobia among a cluster of different countries comprising India, Pakistan, Indonesia and the US, results showed that participants of older ages demonstrated greater levels of resilience (Lindinger-Sternart et al., 2021).

A possible reason for older adults being more resilient could be in their ability to tap on to spiritual activities which has shown to be an efficacious way of dealing with periods of stress. For example, a qualitative study of older adults aged 60 years and above in Singapore, examining the perceptions of social, psychological and physical health identified, among others, that 'the power of prayer' was a common way of coping as placing their concerns regarding their health and emotional worries to a higher power helped them to become more resilient and optimistic (Shiraz et al., 2020).

5.2.2 Understanding religious coping

Turning to God in prayer in times of crisis is not uncommon. A Pew poll (Pew Research Center, 2020) conducted in March 2020 when COVID-19 was declared a global pandemic showed that the virus influenced the religious behaviours of many American adults with more than half of all US adults (55%) saying that they prayed for an end to the pandemic. Of this number, 15% and 24% respectively were among those who seldom or never prayed and those who did not belong to any particular religion. During this same period, the 'Prayer' searches on Google were 50% more than the month before, coinciding with an escalation in the number of infected cases of COVID-19 (Bentzen, 2020).

Pargament et al. (2005) describe religious coping as a process of a person using the religious beliefs and practices of his or her faith to help them cope and deal with stressful moments in one's life. It is a way of coping where the individual is active in interpreting and responding to these stressful life moments (Pargament et al., 2011). Pargament's theory of religious coping includes, among others, elements such as a search for meaning and the sacred, intimacy with others; it is multimodal in that it involves cognitions, emotions, behaviours and relationships, is dynamic in nature and is a process that can lead to both positive or negative outcomes (Pargament et al., 2011).

The Brief Religious Coping Scale (Brief RCOPE) developed by Pargament et al. (1998) identified patterns of religious coping with the following being some examples of positive religious coping: 'seeking spiritual support, collaborative religious coping, spiritual connection, religious purification and benevolent religious reappraisal' (p. 710), while 'spiritual discontent, punishing God reappraisals, interpersonal religious discontent, demonic reappraisal, and reappraisal of God's powers' (p. 710) were examples identified as negative religious coping patterns. These patterns of religious coping have been widely used in studies on stress, crisis, transition and health (Pargament et al., 1998; Pargament et al., 2011).

For example, religious coping has been shown to help older adults deal with difficult situations by relieving tensions and negative emotions in elderly caregivers (Silva et al., 2018), and reducing pain or higher level of acceptance of chronic back pain in older adult patients (Hatefi et al., 2019). Religious coping has also been seen as a mediating factor between religiosity and medication adherence of older adult patients suffering from diabetes as well as improving their overall quality of life (Saffari et al., 2019).

5.2.3 *Religious coping during a pandemic*

Religious coping strategies have been found to be of particular help to deal with the overall worry and anxiety related to the COVID-19 pandemic. Regardless of religious backgrounds and beliefs, positive religious coping strategies seem to positively correlate with positive mental health outcomes. A study among Christians and Muslims in the United Arab Emirates (UAE) on positive religious coping and mental health outcomes as a response to the COVID-19 pandemic showed that for Muslims, positive religious coping was inversely related to depressive symptoms (Thomas & Barbato, 2020). Similarly, results in a study assessing the relationship between religiosity and distress during the pandemic among American Orthodox Jews indicated that there was a strong inverse relationship between positive religious coping and trust in God and stress levels (Pirutinsky et al., 2020). Finally, Lucchetti et al. (2020) notes that there was an increase in the use of religious and spiritual beliefs and practices in an overall sample of Catholics, Evangelicals, Spiritists and even among those who could not report a religion during periods of social isolation due to the pandemic.

5.3 Method

This study employed a phenomenological multiple case study approach and utilised semi-structured interviews as the data collection method. The qualitative approach was more appropriate for this study because the project was intended to be a pilot test for a larger quantitative study in the future. Furthermore, the researchers wanted more in-depth information into a smaller demographic group of older adults. The respondents consisted of nine Catholic older adults, defined as those aged 60 and above according to 2011 Malaysian National Policy for Older Persons (Ministry of Women, Family, and Community Development, 2011), who were identified through the research team's network of contacts.

Purposeful sampling method was used to select the interviewees to ensure gender as well as urban and semi-urban demographic representation. The selected respondents were aged between 64 and 82 years and consisted of three males and six females from the states of Penang, Selangor, Federal Territory of Kuala Lumpur, Terengganu, Johor, Sabah and Sarawak. The research team designed 15 interview questions based on the Brief RCOPE framework for Religious Coping and Well-Being by Pargament et al. (1998). The respondents were asked for their demographic information, the impact of the MCO on their psychological well-being and the methods that they utilised to cope with the situation. As this was a semi-structured interview, members of the research team also asked follow-up questions to elicit more comprehensive explanations and clearer answers.

The research team created an informed consent form which was explained to the participants prior to the interview, and their voluntary consent was obtained before proceeding. Due to restrictions of the pandemic and MCO in Malaysia, interviews with respondents were conducted and recorded via phone or online digital platforms, such as Zoom or Google Meet. Once the interviewees voluntarily agreed to the informed consent form, the interviews were scheduled and conducted by the research team. Strong emphasis was placed on gathering personal narratives, feelings, comments and opinions directly from the older adults. Pseudonyms were used to ensure confidentiality of the respondents' identities. The team of researchers did not have any prior relationship with the interviewees and conducted the interviews separately to avoid bias. Each interview took approximately 45 minutes to an hour. Table 5.1 presents general descriptions of each respondent:

Table 5.1 General description of interview respondents (Catholic older adults)

Pseudonym	Gender	Age
Madam A	Female	64
Madam R	Female	64
Madam AT	Female	82
Mr A	Male	66
Madam J	Female	65
Madam MD	Female	76
Madam RA	Female	65
Mr J	Male	65
Mr AL	Male	64

The interviews were recorded and later transcribed for analysis. The transcriptions were then reviewed and analysed using the constant comparison method and coded through an open coding process (Strauss & Corbin, 1998). Transcriptions were coded line by line in order to identify potential themes that emerged. Coded themes were then categorised based on the Brief RCOPE framework for Religious Coping and Wellbeing by Pargament et al. (1998). Transcriptions were then reviewed again to ensure that the coded themes fitted into the categories described in the theoretical framework.

5.4 Findings and discussion

5.4.1 *Impact on psychological well-being*

Analysis of the data derived from the interviews revealed that Catholic older adults largely experienced increased levels of stress due to fear and anxiety. They also experienced sadness, isolation and loneliness, anger as well as guilt when the MCO was first enforced. However, religious coping strategies helped them to become psychologically resilient and positive-optimistic, hopeful and contented, while feeling grateful and patient; they were also empathetic and kind.

5.4.1.1 *Fear*

Most respondents indicated that they felt scared, afraid and terrified when the pandemic spread and restrictions were imposed. Madam R said, "I was terrified after hearing the news about the virus. It's as if though [sic] we will definitely die once we contract the virus." Madam J expressed similar fears. "I feel quite afraid … middle of March, there was this movement restriction at night from 7pm to 7am … They say it's not a curfew, but we were not supposed to go out, so it kind of dawned on me that it's something so serious that I feel afraid," she said.

5.4.1.2 Sadness and disappointment

The respondents also reported feelings of sadness and disappointment due to the loss of their usual routine, travel ability, family unity and opportunities to physically attend significant life events. Madam RA, for example, said, "I'm not able to go out and that makes me sad ... each time my daughter goes to work, I'll also go out and visit friends. I'll go to market [sic] ... with the pandemic, I'm at home." Furthermore, her routine of physically going to church every Sunday was affected. Said Madam RA, "It was very difficult because ... I never miss church on Sundays ... It was difficult, and it was so strange." Being unable to physically attend Sunday Mass in church resulted in Mr J's sadness about losing family unity and his role as the religious head of his household. Often, only he and his wife attended online Mass as his children were sleepy or preferred to watch on their own. Madam A felt very sad that she was unable to attend her mother's funeral due to travel restrictions.

The respondents' inability to physically receive Holy Communion (*the bread and wine that are given to Catholics who participate at Mass. Catholics believe the bread and wine are the Body and Blood of Jesus as given at the Last Supper*) also contributed to their sadness because online Mass did not fulfil their spiritual needs. Said Madam MD, "Even though spiritually we are receiving the communion, it's nothing like really receiving the Body of Christ." When the respondents were finally able to receive the Sacrament in church, they were overjoyed. Said Madam R, "When I attended physical Mass [sic] after a long time, I cried when I received Holy Communion." Mr J experienced a similar reaction and said, "My tears came out because we were able to receive Holy Communion."

A few respondents were unhappy and dissatisfied with online Masses because they perceived themselves as mere spectators and not participants. Mr J likened online Masses to following a video game or watching a movie where 'we can rewind and playback'. Online Mass did not fulfil his spiritual needs, causing him to feel upset. He said, "... I feel the faith which I had when going to church is ... slowly going down." Madam RA was similarly dissatisfied with online Mass, saying that "we're not participating physically, we're just watching ... There's nothing like being there in person."

5.4.1.3 Anxiety and worry

Overall, there were expressions of anxiety, worry and even paranoia. Madam A said she was anxious because her husband, who is a medical practitioner, is older and has less robust health. The clinic was initially closed, but later reopened albeit with shorter hours. Despite this, Madam A was still worried about exposure to the virus, making her husband bathe as soon as he returned home.

5.4.1.4 Anger and frustration

Some respondents also felt angry, irritable and frustrated. Madam RA felt annoyed that she had to change her habits, such as wearing face masks and washing her hands regularly whenever she went out; changing her clothes and showering after coming home. Madam RA said, "I'm very short tempered now. I get angry fast … I flare up for no reason. I get so annoyed. I want to go here cannot go, there also cannot [sic]. Everywhere you go, have to check temperature [sic], all those things are very annoying." Mr J's quarrels with his wife became more intense as well. Mr J was also upset he was unable to focus during online Mass because his concentration was affected by various distractions around the house.

5.4.1.5 Loneliness and isolation

The respondents also experienced loneliness and isolation because they were unable to meet their family members, relatives and faith community face to face. Mr J said, "We have so many other activities, so when we don't see them together, I feel I'm left out." The loneliness was exacerbated when Mr J was unable to even leave the house for walks and meet with friends and extended family. He said, "Sometimes, I feel very alone. Living alone without anybody listening to us." Madam RA also missed the fellowship with other parishioners. She said, "When we come to church and see all the familiar faces, we miss all that. How many months since I've seen some of my church members. I only speak to them on the phone. It's difficult." Mr AL said that community fellowship cannot be found in online Masses. "I miss the community exchange with other parishioners, so that's why we were very happy when Masses resumed, even with all the restrictions," he added.

5.4.1.6 Guilt

Last, being unable to go for confession led to feelings of guilt by two respondents. Even when face-to-face Masses resumed in church, Madam RA was only able to attend three to four times due to crowd restrictions, which led her to feel she needed to 'ask forgiveness for all the wrong that I've done'. Mr J similarly said, "We haven't done confession for so long, so I feel the faith is going down in that way."

5.4.2 *Minimal negative psychological impact*

Four respondents exhibited minimal negative psychological impact because of their personal circumstances and optimistic disposition. Madam AT did not experience any loss because her son, a Catholic priest, stayed with her, and therefore she received Holy Communion daily. Meanwhile, Madam A, who lived in a semi-urban setting, was used to periods where there was no resident priest to celebrate Mass. She said, "Whenever we had Mass, it was a privilege for us. I learned to treasure that time, so it's not something new actually." Mr A said that his laid-back easy-going outlook enabled him to quickly accept the circumstances, while Mr AL was occupied with his farm work.

5.4.3 *Religious coping strategies: Religious beliefs and practices*

The respondents coped with the psychological impacts by using their religious beliefs and practices. Analysis of data revealed that all respondents expressed use of only positive religious coping strategies. There was no negative religious coping found in the interview responses by these older adults. The patterns of religious coping based on Pargament et al.'s (1998) Brief RCOPE identified in the interview responses will be discussed in the following section.

5.4.4 *Positive religious coping strategies*

The following positive patterns were employed by the older adults interviewed in this study.

5.4.4.1 *Seeking spiritual support and connection through prayer*

The findings showed that the respondents turned to their Catholic faith to weather the challenges of the pandemic. Prayer was a vital element in reaffirming their faith and how they sought spiritual support and connection. All respondents prayed more regularly, for longer durations and with more intensity to get closer to and have a stronger relationship with God. Mr A's prayers became 'lengthier' as he found himself being more 'talkative' with God. Madam A's prayers also increased, and she found herself praying whilst 'washing pots and pans' and doing chores. Madam RA became 'more organised' by waking up at 5am to spend up to 1 hour and 45 minutes praying for family, friends and the whole world. Both Madam R and Madam RA shared that prayer strengthened their faith and helped them deal with fears and challenges.

In addition to personal prayer, respondents also reported an increase in regularity of family prayer time. Madam R and her family prayed the Rosary (*a devotional prayer that makes use of beads to help to reflect on the life of Jesus and His mother, Mary*) together every evening. Mr J and his family also prayed the Rosary and Divine Mercy together (*Divine Mercy is a Catholic devotional prayer that focuses on the mercy of God for humanity*). The respondents also turned to the Bible for spiritual support and connection. Mr J began to read one Bible chapter daily, while Madam RA started reading the Bible 'more in-depth [sic]'. All respondents in this study were found to have used prayer and scripture for more spiritual support and connection.

5.4.4.2 Religious surrender, helping and benevolent appraisal

Surrendering to God's will and performing acts of service were also ways in which the respondents coped with the pandemic. Most respondents found that surrendering to God's will allowed them to count and appreciate their blessings which moved them to help others. Madam RA states that "God has blessed me and I want to bless others back." She also believes that all good deeds are to be done anonymously and echoes this by stating, "that should be the way. I don't want anything in return." Mr AL stated that he fully depended on God to guide him on how to help isolated older adults living alone to access online Mass and connect virtually with the community. He mentioned that "there were a few of them living alone so we try [sic] to keep in touch with them through WhatsApp groups." Madam AT also believed that she is blessed and that the recent life changes made her more patient and generous. Relying on God and focusing on others rather than themselves helped the respondents to cope with the new situation.

5.4.4.3 Seeking religious direction and community support

Church closures during the pandemic disrupted the routine of communal worship and engagement that the respondents had been accustomed to. Many respondents were active members of their parish community who participated in various ministries. The respondents had to look for new ways to cope with the changes caused by the pandemic to their regular faith practices. Among the coping strategies employed was adapting to online Masses and prayer gatherings. The respondents also displayed resourcefulness in seeking various platforms to fulfil their need for spiritual and communal engagement to keep their faith alive and strong.

Although online participation could not offer them the same ambience as worshipping in a physical sacred space, the respondents adapted and even learned to access these online services using their digital devices. They tapped on or created online networks to share information about online Masses, faith-related talks, homilies and fellowship. As a result, their appreciation for online faith resources increased.

These older adults were also able to connect with members of their parish community through online Rosary, prayer groups and their church group living in their neighbourhood. Madam A connected with her community by praying the Rosary together through WhatsApp. Madam RA and her family joined an online chat group and participated in virtual prayer and fellowship where they interacted with other Catholic families. Mr AL joined the Men's Fellowship organised by his diocese which had online activities and discussions such as praise and worship, Bible reflection and a video on men's roles. Although Mr AL preferred face-to-face interactions, participation in a 'spiritual holy communion' and hearing the readings from the Bible did help his spiritual growth. Meanwhile, Mr A, instead of merely participating, also actively used the digital platform to conduct programmes for other Catholics. Such community interactions supported the overall well-being of the older adults.

Respondents also sought religious direction by adapting and becoming resourceful in seeking information to enrich their faith. Madam R discovered various online platforms about the Bible and Sacraments such as 'Logos' and 'Divine' that helped increase her religious knowledge. Mr J used YouTube more frequently during the pandemic to look for religious resources, listen to 'old Catholic songs' and watch 'Gospel movies'. For Mr J, these new media resources have helped deepen his faith. It is evident that the resourcefulness in seeking religious direction online has been a coping tool for the respondents.

5.4.5 Outcome of using positive religious coping strategies

The study found that the positive religious coping strategies employed during the pandemic resulted in the reduction of negative psychological effects on these older adults. These strategies enabled them to reframe their paradigms, be more optimistic, flexible, empathetic and satisfied with their lives. This reframing helped reduce the stress, fears and worries they had to become more resilient and hopeful.

5.4.5.1 Optimism and hope

Most of the respondents revealed optimism and hopefulness that emanated from their strong religious belief and trust in God. Madam J said, "Ya, faith really helped us through this … peculiar time. And I think the Lord is really with us through it all … So thank God." Her husband, Mr A, was also optimistic that the pandemic will be over. He said, "… history tells [sic] that this thing will be over but don't know when … the people will get used to it… but it takes time… we have to wait patiently lah, get the thing to be over [sic]". Mr A added that his Catholic faith gave him 'hope that God is always with us and He will give us the wisdom to overcome this situation' and that 'when the time comes, I will have this communion with God again'.

5.4.5.2 Contentment and satisfaction

The respondents also became more content as they slowly adapted to life under the 'new normal'. Mr A, for example, welcomed the respite from work as the MCO allowed to concentrate on his carpentry hobby. Despite the inconvenience, learning to interact with their faith community via online platforms made Mr A and his wife, Madam J, happy. Mr A found satisfaction in assisting older members to learn digital skills and upgrade their devices. The respondents were also happy to have found faith enrichment through online resources.

5.4.5.3 Empathy, kindness, patience, gratitude

The respondents developed more empathy, kindness and generosity towards the less fortunate. Madam RA said, "This pandemic has taught me to be more caring towards those who're suffering," adding that she has donated to orphanages and old folks' homes. Madam MD displayed empathy when she expressed, "… we don't get anything by complaining … I connect this suffering to your suffering on the cross". The findings also showed that the respondents felt gratitude that their prayer and faith life improved. Madam RA said, "My prayer life has improved and has become stronger. We're all getting old, so have [sic] to get closer to God … Now I have time to go through and mean everything I say. When I pray, I'll talk to God like talking to a friend." These responses by these older adults indicate a reframing of mindset in times of crises to focus on others instead of themselves and be more positive in their outlook.

5.4.6 Negative religious coping

The interview protocol in this study accorded opportunities for respondents to divulge any use of negative religious coping strategies during the pandemic. For example, respondents were asked about their relationship with God and the role their faith has played in their lives during the pandemic. They were also asked to comment about the support received from the Catholic Church and community. However, no negative patterns of religious coping were found.

Analysis of the data revealed that the respondents did not blame God or the Church for the pandemic but instead, they had a very positive outlook about their faith during this time. For example, Madam M does not blame God but instead, feels that "there's a reason God has allowed this pandemic, He didn't bring it but he allowed it for a purpose, so that, you know, maybe we can spend more time with the family." For Mr A, his Catholic faith gave him hope that God is always there and that "He will give us the wisdom to overcome this situation". In his opinion, the Catholic Church in Malaysia has done the best that it could for its community.

5.5 Conclusion

This study reveals that the Catholic older adults initially experienced stress, fear, anxiety and isolation as a result of the pandemic. They experienced these psychological effects due to prolonged separation with family and friends, inability to attend important events and milestones in the family, inability to pray and worship in church and engage with their faith community in person and also due to the disruption to their daily routine inside and outside the home. These findings were consistent with that of Lucchetti et al. (2020) where out of the 485 participants undergoing social isolation (mean = 41.9 days) in the early days of the pandemic in Brazil, 31.5% reported feelings of being very afraid while another 65.2% said that they were very worried as a result of the social isolation.

On the investigation of the religious coping strategies used to deal with the psychological impact of being socially isolated, all respondents in this study employed only positive religious coping methods and were not found to have used negative religious coping methods to effectively manage their psychological well-being during the pandemic. The positive religious coping strategies used include benevolent reappraisals, collaborative religious coping, seeking spiritual support, seeking support from community members, religious helping to others, active religious surrender and seeking spiritual connection (Pargament et al., 1998). These strategies seem to have effectively reduce the negative impact on their psychological well-being as all respondents gradually progressed to feeling more hopeful and resilient in coping with the pandemic.

The findings in this research are aligned with studies such as those by Park et al. (2018) which show that positive religious coping strategies predict higher levels of well-being. Specifically, older adults who have a strong reliance on positive religious coping strategies generally end up with better mental health outcomes when dealing with stressful life events (Pargament et al., 2004; Thomas & Barbato, 2020).

5.5.1 *Limitations of the study*

This study has helped us understand the ways religion expresses itself in the midst of a crisis by identifying particular forms of religious coping that hold significant implications for the psychological well-being of older adults. However, the limitations of this study include the inability to conduct in-person face-to-face interviews and the exclusion of older adults from rural areas who did not have phone or Internet connection. Another limitation was that speakers of other languages were not included as the interviews were conducted in English. Further studies are needed to learn more about the long-term psychological implications of the pandemic and the use of religious coping strategies in times of crisis. This study can be further expanded to include older adults from other faiths, given the multireligious composition of Malaysian society. It would be interesting to identify similarities and differences in terms of the psychological impact and religious coping strategies among Muslims, Hindus, Buddhists and Christians from other denominations. However, this study represents a promising direction for efforts to understand and assist all those who have been impacted by a crisis.

Practical Suggestions

Provide opportunities for small and limited numbers of people on rotation to attend targeted religious services if the space is big enough to allow it. Disseminate information via non-digital mediums like newsletters and flyers to non-technologically savvy persons and those in rural areas. Support social needs by organising small gatherings for communal interactions that adhere strictly to standard operating procedures (SOPs).

References

Archdiocese of Kuala Lumpur Media and Communications Office. (2020, 12th March). Pastoral letter from the Catholic Bishops of Peninsular Malaysia dated 12th March 2020. Suspension of mass and other public gatherings of the faithful in the face of the COVID-19 pandemic. *Archdiocese of Kuala Lumpur.* https://archkl.org/index. php/archkl/archkl-announcement-news/181-march-12-extracts-of-pastoral-letter

Bentzen, J. (2020). *In crisis, we pray: Religiosity and the COVID-19 pandemic* [Unpublished manuscript]. https://www.dropbox.com/s/jc8vcx8qqdb84gn/ Bentzen_religiosity_covid.pdf?dl=0

Hatefi, M., Tarjoman, A., & Borji, M. (2019). Do religious coping and attachment to God affect perceived pain? Study of the elderly with chronic back pain in Iran. *Journal of Religion and Health, 58*(2), 465–475. https://doi.org/10.1007/ s10943-018-00756-9

Koma, W., True, S., Biniek, J. F., Cubanski, J., Orgera, K. & Garfield, R. (2020, October 9). One in four older adults report anxiety or depression amid the COVID-19 pandemic. https://www.kff.org/medicare/issue-brief/one-in-four-older-adults-report-anxiety-or-depression-amid-the-covid-19-pandemic/

Lindinger-Sternart, S., Kaur, V., Widyaningsih, Y., & Patel, A. K. (2021). COVID-19 phobia across the world: Impact of resilience on COVID-19 phobia in different nations. *Counselling and Psychotherapy Research, 21*(2), 290–302. https:// onlinelibrary.wiley.com/doi/10.1002/capr.12387

Lucchetti, G., Góes, L. G., Amaral, S. G., Ganadjian, G. T., Andrade, I., Almeida, P., do Carmo, V. M., & Manso, M. (2020). Spirituality, religiosity, and the mental health consequences of social isolation during Covid-19 pandemic. *The International Journal of Social Psychiatry.* Advance online publication. https:// doi.org/10.1177/0020764020970996

Malaysian Communications and Multimedia Commission (MCMC) (2018). Internet users survey 2018. Statistical brief number twenty-three. https://www.mcmc.gov. my/skmmgovmy/media/General/pdf/Internet-Users-Survey-2018.pdf

Ministry of Women, Family, and Community Development (2011). National Policy for Older Persons. https://fh.moh.gov.my/v3/index.php/component/jdownloads/ send/23-sektor-kesihatan-warga-emas/469-dasar-warga-emas?Itemid=0

Mukhtar, S. (2020). Psychological impact of COVID-19 on older adults. *Current Medicine Research and Practice, 10*(4), 201–202. https://doi.org/10.1016/j. cmrp.2020.07.016

Pargament, K. I., Feuille, M., & Burdzy, D. (2011). The Brief RCOPE: Current psychometric status of a short measure of religious coping. *Religions, 2*(1), 51–76. https://doi.org/10.3390/rel2010051

Pargament, K. I., Koenig, H. G., Tarakeshwar, N., & Hahn, J. (2004). Religious coping methods as predictors of psychological, physical and spiritual outcomes among medically ill elderly patients: A two-year longitudinal study. *Journal of Health Psychology, 9*(6), 713–730. https://doi.org/10.1177%2F1359105304045366

Pargament, K. I., Magyar-Russell, G. M., & Murray-Swank, N. A. (2005). The Sacred and the search for significance: Religion as a unique process. *Journal of Social Issues, 61*, 665–687.

Pargament, K., Smith, B., Koenig, H., & Perez, L. (1998). Patterns of positive and negative religious coping with major life stressors. *Journal for the Scientific Study of Religion, 37*(4), 710–724. https://doi.org/10.2307/1388152

Park, C. L., Holt, C. L., Le, D., Christie, J., & Williams, B. R. (2018). Positive and negative religious coping styles as prospective predictors of well-being in African Americans. *Psychology of Religion and Spirituality, 10*(4), 318–326. https://doi.org/10.1037/rel0000124

Pew Research Center. (2020, March 30). Most Americans say coronavirus outbreak has impacted their lives. https://www.pewsocialtrends.org/2020/03/30/most-americans-say-coronavirus-outbreak-has-impacted-their-lives/

Pirutinsky, S., Cherniak, A. D., & Rosmarin, D. H. (2020). COVID-19, mental health, and religious coping among American Orthodox Jews. *Journal of Religion and Health, 59*(5), 2288–2301. https://doi.org/10.1007/s10943-020-01070-z.

Roupa, Z., Nikas, M., Gerasimou, E., Zafeiri, V., Giasyrani, L., Kazitori, E., & Sotiropoulou, P. (2010). The use of technology by the elderly. *Health Science Journal, 4*, 118.

Saffari, M., Lin, C. Y., Chen, H., & Pakpour, A. H. (2019). The role of religious coping and social support on medication adherence and quality of life among the elderly with type 2 diabetes. *Quality of Life Research: An International Journal of Quality of Life Aspects of Treatment, Care and Rehabilitation, 28*(8), 2183–2193. https://doi.org/10.1007/s11136-019-02183-z.

Shiraz, F., Hildon, Z. L. J., & Vrijhoef, H. J. M. (2020). Exploring the perceptions of the ageing experience in Singaporean older adults: A qualitative study. *Journal of Cross-Cultural Gerontology, 35*, 389–408. https://doi.org/10.1007/s10823-020-09414-8.

Silva, M. C. M., Moreira-Almeida, A., & Castro, E. A. B. (2018). Elderly caring for the elderly: Spirituality as tensions' relief. *Revista Brasileira de Enfermagen, 71*(5), 2461–2468. http://dx.doi.org/10.1590/0034-7167-2017-0370.

Strauss, A., & Corbin, J. (1998). *Basics of qualitative research: Grounded theory procedures and techniques* (2nd ed.). Thousand Oaks, CA: Sage Publications

Thomas, J., & Barbato, M. (2020). Positive religious coping and mental health among Christians and Muslims in response to the COVID-19 pandemic. *Religions, 11*(10), 498–510. http://dx.doi.org/10.3390/rel11100498

World Health Organization (2017, December 12). Mental health of older adults. https://www.who.int/news-room/fact-sheets/detail/mental-health-of-older-adults.

6 Factors promoting university instructor's resilience to technostress

Chia Keat Yap & Si Na Kew

6.1 Introduction

Since the coronavirus disease (COVID-19) pandemic strikes, universities worldwide have shifted to online teaching that emphasises computers and the Internet in providing online education (Alvarez, 2020). However, contrary to conventional online teaching, online teaching during COVID-19 is an emerging approach that put it through during the pandemic outbreak (Trust & Whalen, 2020). This approach is known as "emergency remote teaching" (ERT), and it is described as a temporary shift of instructional mode to an online delivery mode as a result of an unexpected crisis or situation (Trust & Whalen, 2020).

While emergency remote teaching has become the "mainstream" option in most educational institutions, university instructors were found to experience an unprecedented stress level due to the overwhelming demand for computer-mediated technology use in education within a short period (Nambiar, 2020). Experts have warned that inappropriate and excessive use of computers and technology in education could lead to what is known as "technostress", a stressful experience when a person is subjected to information overload and overwhelmed by technology use (La Torre et al., 2019). The term "technostress" was first defined by Brod (1984) as "a modern disease of adaptation caused by the inability to cope with new technologies healthily" (p. 16). Since its inception in the 1980s, technostress has been the central focus in research primarily due to people's concern about how technology can impact individual well-being (Fox et al., 2020).

To better understand technostress, Tarafdar et al. (2007) proposed that there are five relevant technostress creators, namely: (i) techno-overload, related to the strain that arises due to high workload, high pace and prolonged working time in the digital technology environment; (ii) techno-invasion, referring to excessive use of ICT and the obligation to make sure that person is always contactable; (iii) techno-complexity, referring to certain digital

DOI: 10.4324/9781003178576-9

technologies tend to be complicated and ICT workers find it difficult to solve with their existing ICT skills; (iv) techno-insecurity, related to a sense of job insecurity due to high demand in someone highly skilled in ICT and (v) techno-uncertainty, referring to a constant feeling of uncertainty caused by the need to learn and update themselves about ICT continuously. In this chapter, we only measured technostress using three stressors: (i) techno-overload; (ii) techno-invasion and (iii) techno-complexity, as they are relatively relevant in the current scenario where an increase of computer-mediated work is expected and also because of an intensification of remote working.

In Malaysia, Sia and Adamu (2020) found that instructors in higher education institutions encountered various challenges in computer-mediated education, including inadequate infrastructure, lack of experience, low readiness and poor digital literacy. Surprisingly, while studies have documented some techno-stressors encountered by university instructors during the COVID-19 pandemic, no studies have yet to identify factors that can promote resilience among university instructors. Therefore, inattention to this gap may impede understanding of resilience factors that help individuals deal with technostress.

This chapter conceptualises resilience as the ability to bounce back from crises and modify goals and behaviours to cope with changes in the environment (Smith et al., 2010). Resilience in the workplace is a multifaceted construct that can often be studied as either a specific, situational process or a long-lasting stable personality trait (Diehl et al., 2012). Given this, this study will first focus on a relevant domain-specific resilience factor (i.e. computer self-efficacy), followed by two crucial personality traits (i.e. dispositional optimism and self-esteem) to explain the role of resilience in predicting technostress.

In this study, computer self-efficacy is operationalised as an individual's judgement of their ability to use a computer using the Computer Self-Efficacy Scale (CSES). Dispositional optimism is operationalised as the general positive expectancy that positive events are more likely to happen than adverse events across life domains using the Life Orientation Test-Revised (LOT-R). Finally, self-esteem is operationalised as the attitude towards self and the evaluation of the person using the Rosenberg Self-Esteem Scale (RSES).

6.2 Literature review

6.2.1 Computer self-efficacy and technostress

In general, online teaching requires knowledge and skills in using digital devices, particularly computers (Rahim, 2020). One of the resilience factors found to be relevant in this current context is computer self-efficacy. Computer self-efficacy is a domain-specific type of self-efficacy that depicts an individual's judgment of their ability to use a computer (Compeau & Higgins, 1995). Instructor's computer self-efficacy has played a significant role in ICT (Scherer & Siddiq, 2015). For instance, Nambiar (2020) found that computer skill was the main factor for effective online teaching experience. La Paglia et al. (2008) found that teachers with low computer self-efficacy were more susceptible to computer anxiety, a relevant construct with technostress. Celik and Yesilyurt (2013) found that computer self-efficacy was a significant predictor of attitudes towards using computer-supported education. The researchers further explained that individuals with high perceived computer self-efficacy are more confident in computer use, contributing to their positive computer-mediated education experience. In addition, Dong et al. (2020) found that teachers with high self-efficacy were more resilient to technostress. However, studies have yet to be conducted in Malaysia, and thus it is not clear whether such a relationship can be replicated. Nevertheless, based on the previous empirical findings, we hypothesise that:

H1: Computer self-efficacy will negatively predict technostress.

6.2.2 Dispositional optimism and technostress

The COVID-19 pandemic is a crisis that links to many negative psychological consequences, such as negative emotions (i.e. fear) and negative beliefs that the situation can be detrimental and catastrophic (Fofana et al., 2020). Arslan and Yildirim (2020) explained that fear and uncertainty could predispose individuals to become pessimistic about their future during a crisis, which then causes more and feel anxiety and stress. Over the years, experts have advocated that optimistic individuals are more resilient in times of crisis or life transition (Arampatzi et al., 2020). Existing literature often depicts optimism either as a personality trait (i.e. dispositional optimism) or situation-specific (i.e. situational optimism) or domain-specific optimism (e.g. optimism towards computer use).

In this study, we deliberately focused on trait-like optimism (i.e. dispositional optimism) over other types of optimism for two main reasons. First, considering that this study has already focused on a domain-specific resilience factor (i.e. computer self-efficacy), a trait-like optimism becomes crucial. Second, dispositional optimism is considered relatively stable over time compared to other types of optimism (i.e. situation-specific or domain-specific optimism) (Papworth et al., 2019). Dispositional optimism is described as the general positive expectancy that positive events are more likely to happen than adverse events across life domains (Carver & Scheier, 2014). To date, less is known about whether dispositional optimism is predictive of technostress among university lecturers in Malaysia. Nonetheless, based on the previous findings, we hypothesise that:

H2: Dispositional optimism will negatively predict technostress.

6.2.3 Self-esteem and technostress

Self-esteem is defined as the attitude towards self and the evaluation of the person (Rosenberg, 1965). Like dispositional optimism, self-esteem is often considered a personality variable that can help understand how one copes with adversity (Fang et al., 2020). Researchers often called this personality variable "global self-esteem" or "trait self-esteem", and studies have consistently found that self-esteem is another common resilience factor used to study stress (Borji et al., 2020). Self-esteem and stress have been explored with self-esteem functions as the positive appraisal (Chen et al., 2017), for instance, the higher individual's self-esteem, the higher one's evaluation of the ability to cope with a stressor. Therefore, it is expected that instructors with high self-esteem are likely to have a higher evaluation of themselves, which allows them to believe that they can cope with technostress in the current situation. Unfortunately, existing literature and studies in Malaysia have yet to examine whether self-esteem is predictive of technostress. Despite this, a recent study by Korzynski et al. (2020) supported this relationship. The researchers found that self-esteem was negatively associated with technostress levels. Therefore, in our study, we hypothesise that:

H3: Self-esteem will negatively predict technostress.

6.3 Method

6.3.1 Data collection and sample

A cross-sectional correlational research design was employed to understand the prediction of three resilience factors in technostress. The questionnaire was designed using an online Google Form, and the link of the questionnaire was circulated to university lecturers through email and social media webpage. All the participants were informed that their data would be kept confidential and anonymous, and they were presented with a brief explanation of the study's objectives. Moreover, all participants were also informed that their participation in the study was completely voluntary and allowed to leave at any time. To determine the sample size, G*Power software was used to calculate the minimum sample size required. In our study involving three predictors, a medium effect size (0.15) was chosen, and the power

Table 6.1 Demographic profile of respondents (university instructors)

Profile	Frequency (N)	Percentage (%)
Gender		
Male	47	32.6
Female	97	67.4
Ethnicity		
Malays	110	76.4
Chinese	23	16.0
Indians	11	7.6
Others		
Age in years		
20–30	7	4.9
31–40	52	36.1
41–50	53	36.8
51–60	32	22.2
≥ 60		

was set at .80. The calculated minimum sample size required was 77. A convenience sampling method was employed in this study in which all the participants were approached at their convenience time.

The data collection process took approximately 1 month, and initially, there were 145 responses collected. However, one questionnaire set was discarded due to missing info and straightlining. Finally, 144 responses were qualified for data analysis. Table 6.1 shows the demographic information of the participants. Of the total respondents, 32.6% of them were male, and 67.4% were female. In terms of ethnicity, the majority of the participants in the study were Malays (76.4%), followed by Chinese (16.0%) and Indians (7.6%). Besides that, most participants (95.1%) were within the age range of 31–60 years.

6.3.2 Measures

To measure computer self-efficacy, the 12-item CSES was administered (Howard, 2014). The questionnaire is measured on a 7-point scale (from 1 = strongly disagree to 7 = strongly agree), and an example of the item is, "It is easy for me to accomplish my computer goals." The LOT-R was used to measure dispositional optimism (Scheier & Carver, 1992). LOT-R consists of 10-item on a 5-point Likert scale (from 0 = strongly disagree to 4 = strongly agree). The scale contains three positively worded items measuring optimism, for example, "Overall, I expect more good things to happen to me than bad," and three negatively coded items assessing pessimism, for example, "I rarely count on good things happening to me." Another four filler items serve to distinguish the scale purpose.

Although RSES has been previously questioned about its cultural sensitivity (Yeo & Yap, 2020), a recent study supported its application in a multicultural context in Malaysia (Alvani et al., 2021). Therefore, this study used RSES to measure the instructor's self-esteem. RSES is a 10-item questionnaire measured on a 4-point scale (from 1 = strongly agree to 4 = strongly disagree) (Rosenberg, 1965). In total, five positively worded items measure the positive views of one's value, for instance, "I feel that I have a number of good qualities" and another five negatively worded items measure negative views of own value, for example, "All in all, I am inclined to feel that I am a failure." Three technostress creators: (i) techno-overload (4 items), techno-invasion (3 items) and techno-complexity (4 items) (Tarafdar et al., 2007) were chosen to form an 11-item technostress scale to measure technostress. An example of the item for techno-overload is, "I am forced by this technology to work much faster." As for techno-invasion, an example of the item is, "I spend less time with my family due to this technology." Finally, an example of the item for techno-complexity is, "I do not know enough about technology to handle my job satisfactorily." All the items were measured on a Likert scale (from 1 = strongly disagree to 5 = strongly agree).

6.3.3 Data analysis

SPSS version 23 and SmartPLS 3.2.7 software (Ringle et al., 2015) were selected to analyse the data. Since the research goal of the current study is more inclined to the prediction of technostress via three exogenous variables (dispositional optimism, self-esteem and computer self-efficacy), we employed partial least square structural equation modelling (PLS-SEM), as it is suitable for the prediction of key constructs (Hair et al., 2019).

6.3.3.1 Specification of the measurement model

We operationalised all four latent variables employed in the current study as first-order constructs (unidimensional construct), and they were treated as reflective measures. Computer self-efficacy (CSE), dispositional optimism (DO) and self-esteem (SE) were exogenous variables, whereas technostress (TS) was treated as an endogenous variable.

6.3.3.2 Assessment of the measurement model

We assessed the measurement model using convergent validity and discriminant validity. We ascertained the convergent validity by examining the factor loading, average variance extracted (AVE) (Chin, 1998), and composite reliability (CR) (Rahman et al., 2015). Factor loading greater than 0.70 is believed to provide statistical significance and the measurement model fit (Hair et al., 2017). All the items with outer loading less than 0.7 were considered for removal, and those with outer loading less than 0.4 were all removed. In the final decision stage, a total of five items from CSE (1 item), DO (2 items), SE (1 item) and Stress (1 item) were removed from the measurement model. Figure 6.1 indicates the evaluation of the measurement model using PLS-SEM. As indicated in Table 6.2, the composite reliability was above 0.7. This met the suggestion made by Chin (1998) in which the composite reliability should be equal to or at least higher than 0.60 for an exploratory model. AVE describes the average communality for each latent construct in a latent model, and all the AVE values are above 0.50, which is deemed to have adequate convergent validity (Hair et al., 2017).

In this study, we used the Heterotrait Monotrait (HTMT) to assess discriminant validity. Kline (2011) suggested that the HTMT value should be less than 0.85 to establish discriminant validity. As shown in Table 6.3, the HTMT values found in the current study were all less than 0.85.

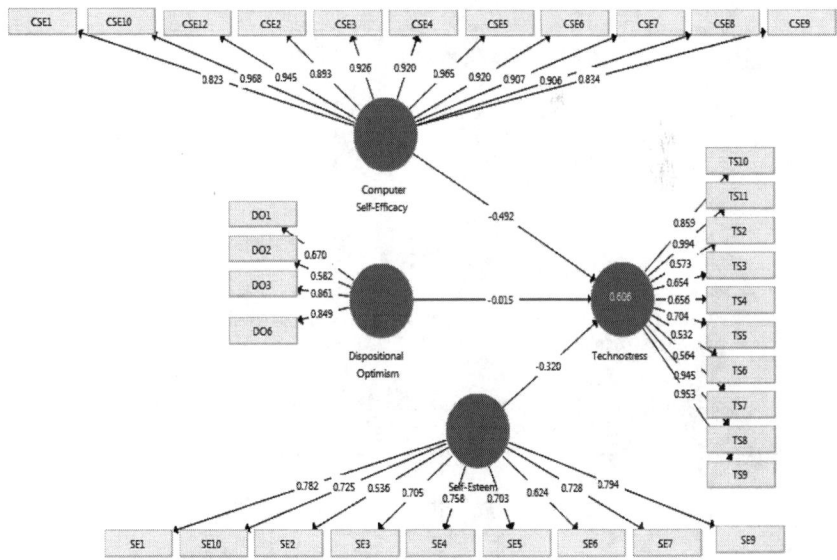

Figure 6.1 The evaluation of measurement model using PLS-SEM.

Table 6.2 Convergent validity of measurement model in PLS-SEM

Construct	Items	Loadings	CR	AVE
Computer self-efficacy (CSE)	CSE1	0.823	0.982	0.829
	CSE2	0.893		
	CSE3	0.926		
	CSE4	0.920		
	CSE5	0.965		
	CSE6	0.920		
	CSE7	0.907		
	CSE8	0.906		
	CSE9	0.834		
	CSE10	0.968		
	CSE12	0.945		
Dispositional optimism (DO)	DO1	0.670	0.834	0.562
	DO2(R)	0.582		
	DO3	0.861		
	DO6	0.849		
Self-esteem (SE)	SE1	0.782	0.901	0.504
	SE2	0.536		
	SE3	0.705		
	SE4	0.758		
	SE5	0.703		
	SE6	0.624		
	SE7	0.728		
	SE9	0.794		
	SE10	0.725		
Technostress (TS)	TS2	0.573	0.930	0.581
	TS3	0.654		
	TS4	0.656		
	TS5	0.704		
	TS6	0.532		
	TS7	0.564		
	TS8	0.945		
	TS9	0.953		
	TS10	0.859		
	TS11	0.994		

Note: CSE11, DO4(R), DO5(R), SE8 and TS1 were deleted due to low loadings. Reversed item is noted with (R).

Table 6.3 Discriminant validity (HTMT ratio) of measurement model in PLS-SEM

	CSE	DO	SE	Technostress
CSE				
DO	0.751			
SE	0.761	0.832		
Technostress	0.731	0.653	0.697	

6.3.3.3 *Evaluation of structural model*

We used the coefficient of determination (R^2), predictive relevance (Q^2), effect size (f^2), path coefficient (β), and t statistic to evaluate our structural model (Hair et al., 2017). The current study showed an average R^2 with a value of 0.606, suggesting that the combination of the three resilience factors explained 60% of the variance in technostress. We computed Stone-Geisser's value (Q^2) to measure the predictive relevance of the structural model. In this study, the observation in our research was 144 and an omission distance of 7 was chosen. The Q^2 value in this study was above 0, suggesting that all the exogenous constructs that were incorporated in the model have predictive relevance (Hair et al., 2017).

6.4 Findings

6.4.1 *Path analyses*

Before proceeding to path analyses, variance inflation factor (VIF) was computed to rule out the possibility of collinearity issues in our study. Essentially, VIF values indicate the extent of correlation between computer self-efficacy, dispositional optimism and self-esteem. Results showed that VIF values of all predictors were below 5, suggesting the absence of collinearity issue in our study. We calculated the path coefficients using the bootstrapping method with a re-sample of 5,000. As shown in Table 6.4, computer self-efficacy ($\beta = -0.492$, $t = 4.801$, $p < 0.01$) and self-esteem ($\beta = -0.320$, $t = 2.216$, $p < 0.05$) negatively predicted technostress, whereas dispositional optimism ($\beta = -0.015$, $t = 0.122$, $p > 0.05$) did not predict stress. Hence, the findings supported H1 and H3, while H2 was not supported. We also computed the effect size (f^2) to understand each resilience factor's impact on technostress. Following the guideline recommended by Cohen (1988), our results showed that computer self-efficacy exerted a moderate effect on stress ($f^2 = 0.225$), whereas self-esteem had a small effect on technostress ($f^2 = 0.066$). However, dispositional optimism did not affect technostress ($f^2 = 0.000$).

Table 6.4 Results of hypothesis testing using PLS-SEM

Hypothesis	Relationship	VIF	Std. Beta	t-value	p values	Decision	f^2
H1	CSE → TS	2.742	−0.492	4.801	0.000	Supported	0.225
H2	DO → TS	3.737	−0.015	0.122	0.903	NS	0.000
H3	SE → TS	3.930	−0.320	2.216	0.027	Supported	0.066

Note: Not supported is denoted as NS.

6.5 Conclusion

Our finding supported our first hypothesis that computer self-efficacy negatively predicted technostress. This finding concurs with previous studies that individuals with higher computer self-efficacy are more resilient to stress (Shu et al., 2011; Tarafdar et al., 2014). The current emergency remote teaching is likely to create extra work demands for university instructors, expecting them to be always available and accessible to their work and posting ongoing challenges computer-mediated technologies problems. Regarding the technology work overload, Shu et al. (2011) found that individuals with higher computer self-efficacy are more resilient than others, and they were able to deal with the mental workload while performing computer-based tasks. Nauta et al. (2009) explained that individuals with low self-efficacy doubt their capability to solve a problem and may experience psychological distress. Moreover, Compeau and Higgins (1995) found that individuals with higher computer self-efficacy are associated with a more positive attitude towards technology use obstacles, allowing them to juggle between work and life. Furthermore, when technology complexities arise, individuals with high computer self-efficacy are less affected as they believe that they have the relevant skills and knowledge in remedying the problems (Tarafdar et al., 2014).

Like the first finding, self-esteem was found to negatively predict technostress, which supports our third hypothesis. Existing literature and empirical findings supported our finding on the relationship between self-esteem and technostress (Juth et al., 2008; Korzynski et al., 2020). Because many lecturers can be overwhelmed by technology workload, invasion of technology and technology complexities, having positive self-esteem is likely to safeguard their sense of self-worth despite facing these technostress creators (Korzynski et al., 2020). Krause et al. (2016) explained that high-self-esteem individuals exhibit more self-confident behaviours, further assisting them in solving various problems. With this in mind, it is reasonable to believe that individuals with positive self-esteem are more resilient and adaptable to ongoing technology-related stressors. Similarly, individuals with high self-esteem are more likely to appraise themselves positively and maintain positive self-attitudes (Kogler et al., 2017), all of which can be useful when confronting technostress.

Contrary to our expectation, our result did not support our second hypothesis as the global optimistic trait was not found to predict technostress. This contradictory finding is likely due to one main reason. Although both dispositional optimism and self-esteem are considered as personality traits in this study, the former focuses on positive expectancies that good things are likely to happen in general while the latter taps into an individual's evaluation of one's overall value, which is closely tied to how one feels about his or her ability to function in a situation. As mentioned earlier, stressors in the current emergency remote teaching often require individuals to believe that they can manage technology-related stressors (Rahim, 2020). Therefore, believing that one can perform computer-related behaviours and feel confident about themselves may seem more useful in tackling technology-related stressors than just being optimistic about the situation.

We also compared the effect sizes to understand the effects of the three exogenous variables (computer self-efficacy, dispositional optimism and self-esteem) on the endogenous variable (technostress). The computer self-efficacy yielded a "moderate" effect on technostress compared to the other predictors (dispositional optimism and self-esteem). Although having been found as another predictor of technostress in this study, self-esteem only contributed to a "small" effect towards technostress. Such finding is likely because computer self-efficacy specifically taps into technology performance beliefs, whereas self-esteem is a global personality trait that measures one's overall self-worth.

6.5.1 *Implications of the study*

This chapter has offered two pivotal implications. First, our non-significant finding on dispositional optimism suggests the need to examine a contextualised variable or variable related to personal ability when studying technostress. More specifically, it is believed that while studying the role of personality traits as resilience factors, one should also focus on personality traits that are at least relevant to personal ability, in our case—self-esteem. Second, our significant findings on computer self-efficacy and self-esteem suggest that training programmes should prioritise bolstering contextual resilience factors that tap into personal ability, in our case the computer self-efficacy, and then followed by a trait-like resilience factor that is relevant to personal ability (i.e. self-esteem). Although having high self-esteem can be pivotal to affirm one sense of worth under adversity, what can be more important is that the lecturer will need to believe that he or she can solve those specific tasks.

6.5.2 *Scope and limitations of the study*

In this study, we were mainly interested in identifying factors that promote the instructor's resilience to technostress. To achieve this, we focused on a domain-specific resilience factor (computer self-efficacy) and two trait-like resilience factors (dispositional optimism and self-esteem). There are a few limitations that should be noted in this study. First, the convenience sampling method employed in the current study limited the generalisability of the findings (Abrams, 2010). Second, causality cannot be inferred due to the cross-sectional nature of this study (Spector, 2019). Therefore, researchers may consider using a longitudinal design for future studies to examine the role of computer self-efficacy and self-esteem as resilience factors over prolonged periods. Third, other variables such as instructors' demographic profiles and their professional backgrounds may affect the relationship between resilience and technostress. Therefore, future studies should consider these variables when examining technostress (e.g. age, gender, teaching experience, expertise, etc.).

Practical suggestions

We recommend that universities provide more workshops that tailor the lecturers' computer self-efficacy (Dong et al., 2020), which can enhance lecturers' ability to tackle technology-related stressors. University management should also organise more psychosocial and interpersonal programmes to enhance lecturers' self-esteem and confidence to cope with technostress.

References

Abrams, L. S. (2010). Sampling "hard to reach" populations in qualitative research: The case of incarcerated youth. *Qualitative Social Work, 9*(4), 536–550. DOI: 10.1177/1473325010367821

Alvani, S. R., Hosseini, S. M. P., Attaran, R., Hashim, I. H., Mohd-Zaharim, N., Selamat, N. H., & Karupiah, P. (2021). Decomposition of gender, self-esteem, social support and family support differentials among university students. *SN Social Sciences, 1*(1), 1–23. DOI: 10.1007/s43545-020-00042-0

Alvarez, A. J. (2020). The phenomenon of learning at a distance through emergency remote teaching amidst the pandemic crisis. *Asian Journal of Distance Education, 15*(1), 127–143. DOI: 10.5281/zenodo.3881529

Arampatzi, E., Burger, M., Stavropoulos, S., & Tay, L. (2020). The role of positive expectations for resilience to adverse events: Subjective well-being before, during and after the Greek bailout referendum. *Journal of Happiness Studies, 21*(3), 965–995. DOI: 10.1007/s10902-019-00115-9

Arslan, G., & Yildirim, M. (2020). Coronavirus stress, meaningful living, optimism, and depressive symptoms: A study of moderated mediation model. *PsyArXiv*, 1–27. DOI: 10.31234/osf.io/ykvzn

Brod, C. (1984). *Technostress: The human cost of the computer revolution.* Reading, MA: Addison-Wesley.

Borji, M., Memaryan, N., Khorrami, Z., Farshadnia, E., & Sadighpour, M. (2020). Spiritual health and resilience among university students: The mediating role of self-esteem. *Pastoral Psychology, 69*(1), 1–10. DOI: 10.1007/s11089-019-00889-y

Carver, C. S., & Scheier, M. F. (2014). Dispositional optimism. *Trends in Cognitive Sciences, 18*(6), 293–299. DOI:10.1016/j.tics.2014.02.003

Celik, V., & Yesilyurt, E. (2013). Attitudes to technology, perceived computer self-efficacy and computer anxiety as predictors of computer supported education. *Computers and Education, 60*(1), 148–158. DOI: 10.1016/j.compedu.2012.06.008

Chen, L., Zhong, M., Cao, X., Jin, X., Wang, Y., Ling, Y., Cen, W., Zhu, X., Yao, S., Zheng, X., & Yi, J. (2017). Stress and self-esteem mediate the relationships between different categories of perfectionism and life satisfaction. *Applied Research in Quality of Life, 12*(3), 593–605. DOI: 10.1007/s11482-016-9478-3

Chin, W. (1998). The partial least squares approach to structural equation modeling. *Modern Methods for Business Research, 295*(2), 295–336. DOI: 10.16/j.aap.2008.12.010

Cohen, J. (1988). *Statistical power analysis for the behavioral sciences* (2nd ed.). Hillsdale, NJ: Erlbaum.

Compeau, D. R., & Higgins, C. A. (1995). Computer self-efficacy: Development of a measure and initial test. *MIS Quarterly, 19*(2), 189–211.

Diehl, M., Hay, E. L., & Chui, H. (2012). Personal risk and resilience factors in the context of daily stress. *Annual Review of Gerontology and Geriatrics, 32*(1), 251–272. DOI:10.1891/0198-8794.32.251

Dong, Y., Xu, C., Chai, C. S., & Zhai, X. (2020). Exploring the structural relationship among teachers' technostress, technological pedagogical content knowledge (TPACK), computer self-efficacy and school support. *Asia-Pacific Education Researcher, 29*(2), 147–157. DOI: 10.1007/s40299-019-00461-5

Fang, M., Li, G., Kang, X., Hou, F., Lv, G., Xu, X., Kong, L., & Li, P. (2020). The role of gender and self-esteem as moderators of the relationship between stigma and psychological distress among infertile couples. *Psychology, Health and Medicine*, 1–14. DOI: 10.1080/13548506.2020.1808233

Fofana, N. K., Latif, F., Sarfraz, S., Bilal, Bashir, M. F., & Komal, B. (2020). Fear and agony of the pandemic leading to stress and mental illness: An emerging crisis in the novel coronavirus (COVID-19) outbreak. *Psychiatry Research*. DOI: 10.1016/j.psychres.2020.113230

Fox, K., Roney, K., & Hargrove, T. (2020). Examining teachers' social emotional status: Effects of covid-19 and technostress. In E. Langran (Ed.), *Proceedings of SITE Interactive 2020 Online Conference* (pp. 469–479). Online: Association for the Advancement of Computing in Education (AACE).

Hair, J., Hollingsworth, C. L., Randolph, A. B., & Chong, A.Y. L. (2017). An updated and expanded assessment of PLS-SEM in information systems research. *Industrial Management and Data Systems, 117*(3), 442–458. DOI: 10.1108/IMDS-04-2016-0130

Hair, J. F., Risher, J. J., Sarstedt, M., & Ringle, C. M. (2019). When to use and how to report the results of PLS-SEM. *European Business Review, 31*(1), 2–24. DOI: 10.1108/EBR-11-2018-0203

Howard, M. C. (2014). Creation of a computer self-efficacy measure: Analysis of internal consistency, psychometric properties, and validity. *Cyberpsychology, Behavior and Social Networking*, 17(10), 677–681. DOI: 10.1089/cyber.2014.0255

Juth, V., Smyth, J. M., & Santuzzi, A. M. (2008). How do you feel? Self-esteem predicts affect, stress, social interaction, and symptom severity during daily life in patients with chronic illness. *Journal of Health Psychology*, 13(7), 884–894. DOI: 10.1177/1359105308095062

Kline, R. B. (2011). *Principles and practice of structural equation modeling* (3rd ed.). NYUS: Guilford Press.

Kogler, L., Seidel, E. M., Metzler, H., Thaler, H., Boubela, R. N., Pruessner, J. C., Kryspin-Exner, I., Gur, R. C., Windischberger, C., Moser, E., Habel, U., & Derntl, B. (2017). Impact of self-esteem and sex on stress reactions. *Scientific Reports*, 7(1), 1–9. DOI: 10.1016/j.yfrne.2019.100796

Korzynski, P., Rook, C., Florent Treacy, E., & Kets de Vries, M. (2020). The impact of self-esteem, conscientiousness and pseudo-personality on technostress. *Internet Research*. DOI: 10.1108/INTR-03-2020-0141

Krause, S., Back, M. D., Egloff, B., & Schmukle, S. C. (2016). Predicting self-confident behaviour with implicit and explicit self-esteem measures. *European Journal of Personality*, 30(6), 648–662. DOI: 10.1002/per.2076

La Paglia, F., Caci, B., & La Barbera, D. (2008). Technostress: A research study about computer self-efficacy, internet attitude and computer anxiety. *Annual Review of Cyber Therapy and Telemedicine*, 6, 61–67.

La Torre, G., Esposito, A., Sciarra, I., & Chiappetta, M. (2019). Definition, symptoms and risk of techno-stress: A systematic review. *International Archives of Occupational and Environmental Health*, 92(1), 13–35. DOI: 10.1007/s00420-018-1352-1

Nambiar, D. (2020). The impact of online learning during COVID-19: students' and teachers' perspective. *The International Journal of Indian Psychology*, 8(2), 783–793. DOI: 10.25215/0802.094

Nauta, A., van Vianen, A., van der Heijden, B., van Dam, K., & Willemsen, M. (2009). Understanding the factors that promote employability orientation: The impact of employability culture, career satisfaction, and role breadth self-efficacy. *Journal of Occupational and Organizational Psychology*, 82(2), 233–251. DOI: 10.1348/096317908X320147

Papworth, S., Thomas, R. L., & Turvey, S. T. (2019). Increased dispositional optimism in conservation professionals. *Biodiversity and Conservation*, 28(2), 401–414. DOI: 10.1007/s10531-018-1665-0

Rahim, A. F. A. (2020). Guidelines for online assessment in emergency remote teaching during the COVID-19 pandemic. *Education in Medicine Journal*, 12(2), 59–68. DOI: 10.21315/eimj2020.12.2.6

Rahman, S. A., Amran, A., Ahmad, N. H., & Taghizadeh, S. K. (2015). Supporting entrepreneurial business success at the base of pyramid through entrepreneurial competencies. *Management Decision*, 53(6), 1203–1223. DOI: 10.1108/md-08-2014-0531

Ringle, C. M., Wende, C. M., & Becker, J.-M. (2015). *Smart PLS 3*. Bönningstedt: SmartPLS GmbH. Retrieved from http://www.smartpls.com

Rosenberg, M. (1965). *Society and the adolescent self-image*. NJ: Princeton University Press

Scheier, M. F., & Carver, C. S. (1992). Effects of optimism on psychological and physical well-being: Theoretical overview and empirical update. *Cognitive Therapy and Research, 16*(2), 201–228. DOI: 10.1007/BF01173489

Scherer, R., & Siddiq, F. (2015). Revisiting teachers' computer self-efficacy: A differentiated view on gender differences. *Computers in Human Behavior, 53*, 48–57. DOI: 10.1016/j.chb.2015.06.038

Shu, Q., Tu, Q., & Wang, K. (2011). The impact of computer self-efficacy and technology dependence on computer-related technostress: A social cognitive theory perspective. *International Journal of Human-Computer Interaction, 27*(10), 923–939. DOI: 10.1080/10447318.2011.555313

Sia, J. K. M., & Adamu, A. A. (2020). Facing the unknown: Pandemic and higher education in Malaysia. *Asian Education and Development Studies, 10*(2), 263–275. DOI: 10.1108/AEDS-05-2020-0114

Smith, B. W., Tooley, E. M., Christopher, P. J., & Kay, V. S. (2010). Resilience as the ability to bounce back from stress: A neglected personal resource? *The Journal of Positive Psychology, 5*(3), 166–176. DOI: 10.1080/17439760.2010.482186

Spector, P. E. (2019). Do not cross me: Optimizing the use of cross-sectional designs. *Journal of Business and Psychology, 34*(2), 125–137. DOI: 10.1007/s10869-018-09613-8

Tarafdar, M., Pullins, E. B., & Ragu-Nathan, T. S. (2014). Technostress: Negative effect on performance and possible mitigations. *Information Systems Journal, 25*(2), 103–132. DOI: 10.1111/isj.12042

Tarafdar, M., Tu, Q., Ragu-Nathan, B. S., & Ragu-Nathan, T. S. (2007). The impact of technostress on role stress and productivity. *Journal of Management Information Systems, 24*(1), 301–328. DOI: 10.2753/MIS0742-1222240109

Trust, T., & Whalen, J. (2020). Should teachers be trained in emergency remote teaching? Lessons learned from the COVID-19 pandemic. *Journal of Technology and Teacher Education, 28*(2), 189–199.

Yeo, K. J., & Yap, C. K. (2020). Helping undergraduate students cope with stress : The role of psychosocial resources as resilience factors. *The Social Science Journal*, 1–23. DOI: 10.1080/03623319.2020.1728501

7 The relationship between emotion regulation and well-being during the pandemic

Resilience as a mediator

Nurul Izzah Fathiah binti Wan Ali Munawar & Eugene Y. J. Tee

7.1 Introduction

The COVID-19 pandemic is an unprecedented global health crisis that has resulted in over 140 million global cases and over 3 million global deaths, as of March 19, 2021 (John Hopkins University, 2021). Countries across the globe have implemented preventive measures to control and contain the spread of COVID-19. These include social distancing, travel restrictions and self-imposed isolation. Despite the necessity of such measures, they exert an immense psychological toll on individuals, leading to reductions in individual well-being (Cerbara et al., 2020). This study examines the use of emotion regulation approaches that could possibly build resilience and contribute to well-being during the pandemic. Specifically, the study examines how reappraisal and suppression influence individuals' resilience and well-being within the context of the COVID-19 pandemic. This work begins with definitions of the variables of interest in the present study before theoretical links between them are built to establish the research question and hypotheses.

Well-being is conceptually defined in this study as a state in which individuals experience effective functioning in both their individual and community life (Lamers et al., 2011). This aligns with the World Health Organization's conceptions of mental health, as "a state of well-being in which the individual realizes their capabilities, can cope with the normal stresses of life, can work productively and fruitfully, and can make a contribution to his or her community" (WHO, 2004, p. 12). Central to this conceptualization of well-being is that the quality of psychological and social support factors also enhances coping and resilience outcomes. When these support factors are threatened due to the pandemic,

DOI: 10.4324/9781003178576-10

individuals may face a wide range of different, unpleasant emotions. This is in part due to challenges faced in effectively managing emotions such as loneliness, depression, anxiety and stress (Otu et al., 2020; Wong et al., 2021). As such, it is critical to examine the psychological factors that promote resilience and well-being during the ongoing COVID-19 pandemic.

Emotion regulation are automatic or controlled conscious processes that determine (i) what emotions individuals experience, (ii) when they experience them and (iii) how these emotions are experienced and expressed (Gross, 2001). Through effective, adaptive emotion regulation, individuals are able to deal with daily obstacles and challenges in hopes of well-being maintenance and enhancement (Kalisch et al., 2019). Healthy emotion regulation has been shown to contribute to enhanced resilience (Cano et al., 2020).

Resilience is defined as one's adaptive way of handling stressful events that maintains their physical and psychological strength and well-being (Campbell-Sills & Stein, 2007). Resilience entails an individual's capacity for the continued pursuit of goals and progression towards a positive future despite experienced hardships (Campbell-Sills & Stein, 2007). Studies show that resilient individuals are better able to rebound from stressful events, assert control over their circumstances, and tap into positive emotional resources to buffer against the effects of negative emotions (Restubog et al., 2020).

7.2 Literature review

7.2.1 *Process model of emotion regulation*

Gross' (2001) process model categorises emotion regulation approaches as either antecedent-, cognitive- or response-focused strategies. Antecedent-focused strategies include situation selection and situation modification, wherein individuals attempt to regulate emotions by avoiding or altering the situation eliciting the emotional response in the first place. Attentional deployment and cognitive change are cognitive-focused approaches, which relate to regulating attention and modification of one's appraisal of the situation. Finally, individuals may choose response modulation—attempting to regulate emotional experiences following the incident. Questions remain, however, on how different approaches to emotion regulation help individuals deal with negative emotional experiences, particularly those felt during the COVID-19 pandemic.

Two emotion regulation strategies that have been the subject of some research in this regard are cognitive reappraisal (a cognitive-focused strategy) and expressive suppression (a response-focused strategy). The rationale for focusing on cognitive reappraisal and expressive suppression for this study is twofold. First, numerous studies across cultures conceptualise these two approaches as 'opposites' in how individuals attempt to modify their emotional experiences. Reappraisal and suppression are thus conceptually distinct and commonly used approaches by individuals to regulate their emotions. Differentiating the effects of these two approaches will allow the present study to assess how each affects Malaysians' well-being. Second, given that respondents are unlikely able to pre-empt or avoid emotions associated with the pandemic, antecedent-focused approaches would be deemed unsuitable or unfeasible during this time. In short, the justification for these two strategies is based on theoretical and practical grounds.

7.2.1.1 Cognitive reappraisal

Cognitive reappraisal involves a change in perception about an event to reduce its emotional impact. This approach has been found to help individuals adapt to their stressful situations by allowing them to upregulate positive emotions and downregulate negative emotions (Gross, 2015). By reappraising or reinterpreting the emotion-eliciting incident, the individual attempts to view the situation and circumstances in a more balanced, objective and holistic manner. Reappraisal has generally been shown to be an adaptive and healthy approach to regulating emotions (McRae, 2016). The approach has also been found to help in maintaining social and emotional well-being (Chervonsky & Hunt, 2017). Verzeletti et al. (2016) noted that reappraisal leads to healthier emotional patterns, better social functioning and well-being as compared to suppression. Reappraisal also generates positive emotions that enhance well-being (Nezlek & Kuppens, 2008).

7.2.1.2 Expressive suppression

Expressive suppression involves the inhibition of emotion-expressive behaviour(s). While this approach does result in a reduction of negative emotional expressions, it may potentially cause the experienced negative emotions to linger and remain unresolved (Gross, 2015). The use of suppression results in individuals directing their cognitive resources towards containing their emotions. This contrasts with reappraisal, where efforts and resources are directed instead towards a revaluation of one's circumstances. Studies indicate that reappraisal, but not suppression, aids in the regulation of unpleasant, challenging emotions (Kalokerinos et al., 2015).

Puente-Martínez et al. (2018) showed that suppression leads to diminished emotional and psychological well-being. Moti et al. (2020) find that since suppression involves individuals avoiding and compartmentalising their emotions in hopes of coping with them, they would experience less ownership and control over their emotions. Ultimately, this lowers individuals' perceived competence in managing their emotions and in regulating them for enhanced well-being.

Studies indicate that individuals often use suppression to deal with daily stressors (Cameron & Overall, 2018). This, however, leads to adverse mental health outcomes such as greater depressed mood and lowered life satisfaction. Further, findings also indicate that the use of suppression results in diminished relationship quality. This finding is important in informing our following hypothesis. Despite some claims that suppression of negative and unpleasant emotions may be beneficial—even culturally appropriate when confronting stressful situations (e.g. De Vaus et al., 2018), the current COVID-19 pandemic is a novel existential threat where suppression is likely to be detrimental to well-being. Engaging in suppression in the current circumstances may exacerbate, rather than attenuate, individual well-being. This is because, in addition to imposed self-isolation and the need to comply with strict social and physical distancing measures, suppression would limit opportunities for individuals to meaningfully connect and relate with others, diminishing their well-being. Evidence for this claim is further based on Chervonsky and Hunt's (2017) meta-analysis, indicating that suppression of emotions leads to poorer social well-being and satisfaction, as well as lower perceived social support.

7.2.2 The relationship between emotion regulation and resilience

Effective emotion regulation approaches (i.e. reappraisal) can be considered a crucial personal resource for building resilience (Crane et al., 2019), aiding individuals to cope healthily with adverse emotional events. Georgoulas-Sherry (2020) proposes that individuals who engage in reappraisal effectively balance both positive and negative emotional experiences. Individuals who engage in reappraisal have also been shown to be more accepting, mindful and non-reactive towards their experience of negative emotions relative to those who engage in suppression (Iani et al., 2019). Crucially, these individuals also develop a stronger sense of core beliefs, eventually leading to enhanced self-efficacy and problem-solving capabilities (Luu, 2021).

Clear links are observed between reappraisal and resilience in recent research. Thomas and Zolkoski (2020), for example, found that individuals' resilience increased as a result of using reappraisal. Mouatsou and Koutra (2021) found that resilience was positively associated with reappraisal and negatively associated with suppression. Importantly, such perceptions and beliefs are likely to be influenced by reappraising situations as challenging, instead of simply threatening. In this regard, individuals who reappraise their experiences in light of the COVID-19 pandemic as challenging instead of threatening are more likely to report higher levels of resilience. Further, studies on stress appraisal show individuals who evaluate their stress experiences as challenges are more likely to engage in approach-oriented (rather than avoidance-oriented) behaviours. Ultimately, this leads these individuals to respond more proactively and optimally to their challenges (Jamieson et al., 2018). Given the evidence, it seems reasonable to propose that reappraisal will lead to individuals reporting higher levels of resilience. Conversely, suppression should be negatively associated with resilience. Using suppression to regulate emotions may lead to an unhealthy build-up of negative emotions and depletion of cognitive resources, ultimately diminishing resilience. The first two hypotheses are:

H1: There will be a positive relationship between reappraisal and resilience.
H2: There will be a negative relationship between suppression and resilience.

7.2.3 The relationship between resilience and well-being

The COVID-19 pandemic underscores the importance of resilience in promoting well-being. Numerous studies, employing data collected during the pandemic across different countries and cultures indicate a positive association between resilience and well-being (Kimhi et al., 2020; Prime et al., 2020). Paredes et al. (2021) found that resilient individuals were less affected by the anxieties and stress brought about by the pandemic, while Nitschke et al. (2020) found that greater social connectedness was associated with greater resilience and reduced COVID-19 fatigue. Shanahan et al. (2020) examined resilience factors among young adults during the pandemic, finding that individuals who used more active and healthy coping strategies (e.g. positive reappraisal and reframing) were more likely to report lower levels of perceived stress and anger. Resilient individuals may thus have a more positive perception of their ability to maintain their well-being through pursuing goals that bring a sense of control and meaning into their lives. These goals could include ensuring access to daily necessities, taking care of one's health and that of others amid the pandemic. The research evidence shows a clear link between resilience and well-being, and justifies the following hypothesis:

> H3: There will be a positive relationship between resilience and well-being.

7.2.4 Mediating effect of resilience

The review implies that resilience explains the relationship between emotion regulation and well-being. As such, the relationships between these variables suggest that whether individuals' emotion regulation leads to enhanced well-being depends on the approach they take. Individuals who engage in reappraisal are likely to be more resilient, leading them to also report elevated levels of well-being. Conversely, individuals engaging in suppression will report diminished levels of well-being, as a consequence of lowered perceptions of their resilience. In this instance, diminished resilience serves as the key underlying mechanism linking suppression with lowered well-being. Thus, it is hypothesized that:

> H4: Resilience mediates the relationship between reappraisal and well-being.
> H5: Resilience mediates the relationship between suppression and well-being.

7.2.5 Research question and expected contributions

The research question is, "Does resilience mediate the relationships between emotion regulation strategies and well-being among Malaysians amidst the COVID-19 pandemic?" Results of the current study could potentially highlight the importance of the contributions emotional regulation approaches have towards resilience and subsequently, individual well-being within the context of the COVID-19 pandemic (Killgore et al., 2020). Specifically, results could indicate the underlying mechanisms by which effective emotional regulation approaches cultivate individual well-being. The current study's findings could also provide insight into emerging literature on the importance of understanding differences in emotional regulation approaches amidst the pandemic within an Asian context, along with the importance of cultivating resilience during this time (Bryce et al., 2020).

7.3 Method

7.3.1 Research design

The present study employed a non-experimental correlational design with two predictor variables (reappraisal and suppression), one mediator (resilience), and one outcome variable (well-being). Data were collected through an online survey.

7.3.2 Sample

One hundred (100) Malaysians aged 18–60 years ($M = 28.25$, $SD = 11.56$) responded to an online survey. The majority of respondents were female ($n = 84$). The sample meets the recommended sample size required to detect medium effect sizes ($f^2 = 0.15$) at an alpha level of 0.05 and achieve a power of 0.80. Respondent recruitment was conducted through convenience and snowball sampling.

7.3.3 Measures

7.3.3.1 Emotion regulation

Emotion regulation was measured using the 10-item Emotion Regulation Questionnaire (ERQ; Gross & John, 2003). The measure assesses an individual's tendency of employing reappraisal and suppression to regulate their emotions. An example item for reappraisal is, "When I'm faced with a stressful situation, I make myself think about it in a way that helps me stay calm." An example item for expressive suppression is, "When I am feeling negative emotions, I make sure not to express them." This measure was scaled on a 7-point Likert scale ranging from 1 (*Strongly disagree*) to 7 (*Strongly agree*). Gross and John (2003) report the items to be reliable at $\alpha = 0.79$ for reappraisal and 0.73 for suppression.

7.3.3.2 Resilience

Resilience was measured using the 10-item Connor-Davidson Resilience Scale (CD-RISC; Campbell-Sills & Stein, 2007). The CD-RISC asks individuals whether statements such as, "tend to bound back after illness or hardship" and "not easily discouraged by failure" accurately describe them. This measure is scaled on a 5-point Likert scale ranging from 0 (*Not true at all*) to 4 (*True nearly all the time*). Campbell-Sills and Stein (2007) report this measure to be reliable at $\alpha = 0.85$.

7.3.3.3 Well-being

Well-being was measured using 11 items from the Mental Health Continuum-Short Form (MHC-SF; Lamers et al., 2011). Despite being labelled a mental health measure, the MHC-SF assesses psychological and social well-being. Lamers and colleagues operationalise the MHC-SF as a measure of positive mental health and well-being, instead of mental illness. This measure asks respondents the frequency to which they report feeling positive experiences indicative of elevated social well-being ("I had something important to contribute to society") and psychological well-being ("I think my life has a sense of direction or meaning to it"). Items were scaled on a 6-point Likert scale ranging from 1 (*Never*) to 6 (*Everyday*). Lamers et al. (2011) report this measure to be reliable at $\alpha = 0.89$.

7.3.4 Procedure

Participants were invited to complete the study via an online survey link. After being briefed on the study's details, they provided consent to participate in the study and proceeded to complete the questionnaires. Upon completion, participants were thanked and asked to forward the survey link to anyone they know, between the ages of 18 and 60. The survey was open to all Malaysians and did not impose gender, ethnicity requirements. Data was collected from November to December 2020.

7.3.5 Statistical analysis approach

A series of multiple linear regression and mediation analyses were employed using JASP version 0.14.0.0 to test the hypotheses, given that all data were continuous variables.

7.4 Findings

7.4.1 Descriptive statistics and scale reliabilities

Descriptive statistics and scale reliabilities of all variables are presented on the bivariate correlation table. Table 7.1 also indicates that all measures reliable at $\alpha = 0.76$ and greater.

7.4.2 Assumption tests

Given the modest sample for this study, key assumptions were assessed before conducting the hypothesis tests. The data met assumptions of

Table 7.1 Bivariate correlation table for reappraisal, suppression, resilience and well-being

	M	S.D.	1	2	3	4	5	6
1. Gender	1.86	.38						
2. Age	28.25	11.56	−0.17					
3. Reappraisal	5.44	1.05	−0.12	0.23[a]	(0.83)			
4. Suppression	4.45	1.35	0.04	0.05	0.19	(0.76)		
5. Resilience	2.76	0.65	−0.10	0.33[b]	0.53[b]	0.02	(0.86)	
6. Well-being	3.15	1.00	−0.08	0.33[b]	0.47[b]	−0.01	0.61[b]	(0.91)

Note: Values in bold and in brackets represent the measure's reliability. Gender: 1 = Male; 2 = Female (Dummy-coded).

[a] $p < 0.05$
[b] $p < 0.001$.

normality with the Shapiro-Wilk test indicating that the data did not significantly depart from normality, $W(100) = 0.99$, $p = 0.878$. The data also met the assumption of independence of errors (Durbin-Watson value = 2.15). It was also observed that the data met assumptions of homoscedasticity from the scatterplot of standardised residual values. Finally, there was no indication of multicollinearity, with the variance inflation factor (VIF) for all variables at 1.31 and lower. The results of these assumption tests suggest the suitability of the regression analyses for this data. It was also found that there were no gender differences in any of the focal variables. Age, however, was associated with reappraisal, resilience and well-being at $r = 0.23$ ($p < 0.05$) and greater and was thus controlled for in the analyses.

7.4.3 Hypothesis tests

7.4.3.1 Main effect hypotheses (H1–H3)

Age was controlled for in all main effect tests given its significant relationship with resilience and well-being. We entered age in Step 1 of the regression analyses before the inclusion of resilience in all analyses. Regression analyses showed that reappraisal was significantly associated with resilience, $\beta = 0.41$, $p < 0.001$, supporting H1. Suppression, however, was not a significant predictor of resilience, $\beta = 0.02$, $p = 0.810$. H2 is not supported. The results also indicate that controlling for age, resilience significantly predicts well-being, $\beta = 0.53$, $p < 0.001$, supporting H3.

Table 7.2 Tests of hypothesised mediating effects of resilience on the relationships between reappraisal and well-being, and between suppression and well-being

Indirect effect	Estimate	Standard error	z-value	p	95% Confidence interval	
					Lower	Upper
Reappraisal → Resilience → Well-being	0.177	0.052	3.417	0.000	0.094	0.287
Suppression → Resilience → Well-being	−0.025	0.037	−0.670	0.503	−0.110	0.064

7.4.3.2 Mediating hypotheses (H4 and H5)

Mediation analyses were conducted to test for the potential mediating effect of resilience in explaining emotion regulation and well-being's link, with age as a control in these analyses. The indirect effect of reappraisal on well-being through resilience was significant, based on a bias-corrected bootstrapped confidence interval based on 5,000 bootstrap samples. The 95% confidence interval of this effect [0.094, 0.287] does not contain a zero, indicating that mediation occurred. Results provide support for H4, indicating that reappraisal promotes well-being through elevated levels of resilience. It was then tested if resilience mediated the suppression-well-being link. The 95% biased-corrected bootstrap confidence interval for the indirect effect of suppression on well-being [−0.110, 0.064] contains a zero, indicating the absence of a mediating effect. No support is found for H5. Results of the mediating effects are shown in Table 7.2.

The path plot depicting the tested model and coefficients for the three paths (a, b and c') are depicted in Figure 7.1.

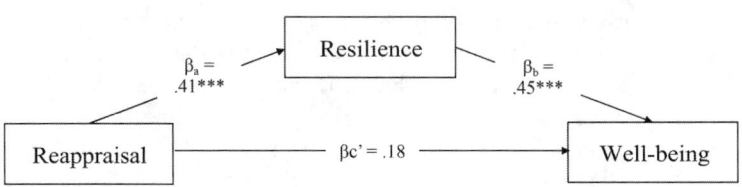

Figure 7.1 Path plot of the significant indirect effect of reappraisal on well-being through resilience.

7.5 Conclusion

7.5.1 The summary of findings

The current study examined resilience's mediating role in the relationship between emotion regulation and well-being among Malaysians during the COVID-19 pandemic. Five hypotheses were proposed based on the use of two emotion regulation strategies—reappraisal and suppression. Mediation analyses were conducted to assess whether the effects of these emotion regulation approaches were associated with well-being via resilience's indirect effect. The results showed that reappraisal and resilience were both significantly and positively associated with well-being. Resilience mediated the relationship between reappraisal and well-being but did not mediate the relationship between suppression and well-being. The results of the study also show that suppression is not significantly associated with either resilience or well-being, aligning with research that generally shows this approach to emotion regulation as non-significant or as a negative influence on desirable psychological outcomes (Chervonsky & Hunt, 2017). To the best of our knowledge, our study is also one of the first to assess what Malaysians actively do to regulate their emotions and manage their well-being during the pandemic compared to the bulk of studies during this period which only assessed the psychological and psychosocial consequences of the pandemic (Yunus et al., 2020).

7.5.2 Limitations of the study and recommendations for future research

Despite the significant results, future studies should examine whether emotion regulation approaches—beyond that of reappraisal and suppression, also enhance resilience and well-being. Future studies should also assess whether respondents who employ attentional re-deployment (e.g. mindfulness meditation), report higher levels of resilience and well-being.

Second, future studies should also consider individual differences that shape the underlying motives for emotion regulation. When regulating their emotions, individuals are inherently motivated to obtain hedonic or instrumental benefits (Ortner et al., 2018). Future studies should uncover motives that could help further understand the influences on individuals' choice of strategies that are perceived most effective in managing their emotions, and whether these also predict resilience and well-being. Further, studies comparing demographic differences will be important given the largely female sample in the study, which limits the generalisability of the current study.

Third, we acknowledge that the cross-sectional design of the study provides a static representation of how Malaysians regulate their emotions. As such, the current study is limited in that it provides just a snapshot of Malaysians' resilience and well-being—during the second wave of the pandemic. Future studies can nonetheless use the current findings and data and compare them with data collected at a different time point. Such comparisons can thus highlight fluctuations in resilience and well-being over time and form the basis for longitudinal designs.

7.5.3 Theoretical implications

The present study's results are consistent with findings from Chervonsky and Hunt (2017) and Verzeletti et al. (2016), who found that reappraisal increased one's well-being. The current study's findings showed that when individuals used reappraisal, the more likely they are to report increased well-being. This dovetails with the literature showing that reappraisal is a healthy and adaptive emotion regulation approach that builds resilience (McRae, 2016). Suppression was not associated with resilience, complementing past studies that have either found a negative or non-significant relationship between the two variables (Mouatsou & Koutra, 2021).

The pattern of results is broadly consistent with claims that reappraisal is beneficial to resilience building, as compared to suppression (Johnson et al., 2017). The findings more broadly contribute to research on psychological factors promoting resilience in non-Western samples. Employing a Malaysian sample for this study, findings from this study contribute to the need to understand resilience factors across different cultural contexts (Ungar & Theron, 2020) and complement studies showing that resilience is a protective factor against adverse mental health outcomes (Brailovskaia et al., 2018). The current study also shows that within the context of the COVID-19 pandemic and in a collectivist culture such as Malaysia, reappraisal is more adaptive in contributing to resilience and well-being than suppression. The findings also contribute to scant research on the psychological factors that promote or inhibit resilience within the Malaysian context amidst the COVID-19 pandemic. Results of the present study complement emerging efforts to understand psychological factors that aid in Malaysians' recovery and resilience during these challenging circumstances (Tee et al., 2021). In the case of the present study, it is shown how healthy, effective regulation of one's emotions, via reappraisal, builds resilience and enhances well-being among Malaysians during this unprecedented health crisis.

Practical suggestions

Mental health professionals may use these findings to suggest that clients re-evaluate their emotion regulation strategies and engage in more adaptive emotion regulation approaches for enhanced resilience and well-being during the pandemic. Individuals may cultivate expressive writing (Pennebaker & Smyth, 2016) as a healthy way to reappraise their emotional experiences.

References

Brailovskaia, J., Schönfeld, P., Zhang, X. C., Bieda, A., Kochetkov, Y., & Margraf, J. (2018). A cross-cultural study in Germany, Russia, and China: Are resilient and social supported students protected against depression, anxiety, and stress?. *Psychological Reports, 121*(2), 265–281. https://doi.org/10.1177/0033294117727745

Bryce, C., Ring, P., Ashby, S., & Wardman, J. K. (2020). Resilience in the face of uncertainty: Early lessons from the COVID-19 pandemic. *Journal of Risk Research, 23*(7–8), 880–887. https://doi.org/10.1080/13669877.2020.1756379

Cameron, L. D., & Overall, N. C. (2018). Suppression and expression as distinct emotion-regulation processes in daily interactions: Longitudinal and meta-analyses. *Emotion, 18*(4), 465–480. https://doi.org/10.1037/emo0000334

Campbell-Sills, L., & Stein, M. B. (2007). Psychometric analysis and refinement of the Connor-Davidson resilience scale (CD-RISC): Validation of a 10-item measure of Resilience. *Journal of Traumatic Stress, 20*(6), 1019–1028. https://doi.org/10.1002/jts.20271

Cano, M., Castro, F. G., De La Rosa, M., Amaro, H., Vega, W. A., Sánchez, M., Rojas, P., Ramírez-Ortiz, D., Taskin, T., Prado, G., Schwartz, S. J., Córdova, D., Salas-Wright, C. P., & de Dios, M. A. (2020). Depressive symptoms and resilience among Hispanic emerging adults: Examining the moderating effects of mindfulness, distress tolerance, emotion regulation, family cohesion, and social support. *Behavioral Medicine, 46*(3–4), 245–257. https://doi.org/10.1080/08964289.2020.1712646

Cerbara, L., Ciancimino, G., Crescimbene, M., La Longa, F., Parsi, M. R., Tintori, A., & Palomba, R. (2020). A nation-wide survey on emotional and psychological impacts of COVID-19 social distancing. *European Review for Medical and Pharmacological Sciences, 24*(12), 7155–7163. https://doi.org/10.26355/eurrev_202006_21711

Chervonsky, E., & Hunt, C. (2017). Suppression and expression of emotion in social and interpersonal outcomes: A meta-analysis. *Emotion, 17*(4), 669–683. https://doi.org/10.1037/emo0000270

Crane, M. F., Searle, B. J., Kangas, M., & Nwiran, Y. (2019). How resilience is strengthened by exposure to stressors: The systematic self-reflection model of resilience strengthening. *Anxiety, Stress, & Coping, 32*(1), 1–17. https://doi.org/10.1080/10615806.2018.1506640

De Vaus, J., Hornsey, M. J., Kuppens, P., & Bastian, B. (2018). Exploring the East-West divide in prevalence of affective disorder: A case for cultural differences in coping with negative emotion. *Personality and Social Psychology Review, 22*(3), 285–304. https://doi.org/10.1177/1088868317736222

Georgoulas-Sherry, V. (2020). Expressive flexibility and resilience among U.S. Military college students: Evaluating the enhancing and suppressing of emotions and resilience. *Journal of Positive School Psychology, 4*(2), 187–198. https://doi.org/10.47602/jpsp.v4i2.225

Gross, J. J. (2001). Emotion regulation in adulthood: Timing is everything. *Current Directions in Psychological Science, 10*(6), 214–219. https://doi.org/10.1111/1467-8721.00152

Gross, J. J. (2015). The extended process model of emotion regulation: Elaborations, applications, and future directions. *Psychological Inquiry, 26*(1), 130–137. https://doi.org/10.1080/1047840X.2015.989751

Gross, J. J., & John, O. P. (2003). Individual differences in two emotion regulation processes: Implications for affect, relationships, and well-being. *Journal of Personality and Social Psychology, 85*(2), 348–362. https://doi.org/10.1037/0022-3514.85.2.348

Iani, L., Lauriola, M., Chiesa, A., & Cafaro, V. (2019). Associations between mindfulness and emotion regulation: The key role of describing and nonreactivity. *Mindfulness, 10*(2), 366–375. https://doi.org/10.1007/s12671-018-0981-5

Jamieson, J. P., Crum, A. J., Goyer, J. P., Marotta, M. E., & Akinola, M. (2018). Optimizing stress responses with reappraisal and mindset interventions: An integrated model. *Anxiety, Stress, & Coping, 31*(3), 245–261. https://doi.org/10.1080/10615806.2018.1442615

John Hopkins University (2021, March 19). COVID-19 Dashboard by the Center for Systems Science and Engineering (CSSE) at Johns Hopkins University (JHU). https://www.arcgis.com/apps/opsdashboard/index.html#/bda7594740fd40299423467b48e9ecf6

Johnson, J., Panagioti, M., Bass, J., Ramsey, L., & Harrison, R. (2017). Resilience to emotional distress in response to failure, error or mistakes: A systematic review. *Clinical Psychology Review, 52*, 19–42. https://doi.org/10.1016/j.cpr.2016.11.007

Kalisch, R., Cramer, A. O. J., Binder, H., Fritz, J., Leertouwer, I., Lunansky, G., Meyer, B., Timmer, J., Veer, I. M., & van Harmelen, A.-L. (2019). Deconstructing and reconstructing resilience: A dynamic network approach. *Perspectives on Psychological Science, 14*(5), 765–777. https://doi.org/10.1177/1745691619855637

Kalokerinos, E. K., Greenaway, K. H., & Denson, T. F. (2015). Reappraisal but not suppression downregulates the experience of positive and negative emotion. *Emotion, 15*(3), 271–275. https://doi.org/10.1037/emo0000025

Killgore, W. D. S., Taylor, E. C., Cloonan, S. A., & Dailey, N. S. (2020). Psychological resilience during the COVID-19 lockdown. *Psychiatry Research, 291*. https://doi.org/10.1016/j.psychres.2020.113216

Kimhi, S., Marciano, H., Eshel, Y., & Adini, B. (2020). Recovery from the COVID-19 pandemic: Distress and resilience. *International Journal of Disaster Risk Reduction, 50*, 101843. https://doi.org/10.1016/j.ijdrr.2020.101843

Lamers, S. M. A., Westerhof, G. J., Bohlmeijer, E. T., ten Klooster, P. M., & Keyes, C. L. M. (2011). Evaluating the psychometric properties of the mental health continuum-short form (MHC-SF). *Journal of Clinical Psychology, 67*(1), 99–110. https://doi.org/10.1002/jclp.20741

Luu, T. T. (2021). Worker resilience during the COVID-19 crisis: The role of core beliefs challenge, emotion regulation, and family strain. *Personality and Individual Differences, 179*, 110784. https://doi.org/10.1016/j.paid.2021.110784

McRae, K. (2016). Cognitive emotion regulation: A review of theory and scientific findings. *Current Opinion in Behavioral Sciences, 10*, 119–124. https://doi.org/10.1016/j.cobeha.2016.06.004

Moti, B., Benish-Weisman, M., Matos, L., & Torres, C. (2020). Integrative and suppressive emotion regulation differentially predict well-being through basic need satisfaction and frustration: A test of three countries. *Motivation and Emotion, 44*(1), 67–81. https://doi.org/10.1007/s11031-019-09781-x

Mouatsou, C., & Koutra, K. (2021). Emotion regulation in relation with resilience in emerging adults: The mediating role of self-esteem. *Current Psychology.* https://doi.org/10.1007/s12144-021-01427-x

Nezlek, J. B., & Kuppens, P. (2008). Regulating positive and negative emotions in daily life. *Journal of Personality, 76*(3), 561–580. https://doi.org/10.1111/j.1467-6494.2008.00496.x

Nitschke, J. P., Forbes, P. A. G., Ali, N., Cutler, J., Apps, M. A. J., Lockwood, P. L., & Lamm, C. (2020). Resilience during uncertainty? Greater social connectedness during COVID-19 lockdown is associated with reduced distress and fatigue. *British Journal of Health Psychology, 26*(2), 553–569. https://doi.org/10.1111/bjhp.12485

Ortner, C. N. M., Corno, D., Fung, T. Y., & Rapinda, K. (2018). The roles of hedonic and eudaimonic motives in emotion regulation. *Personality and Individual Differences, 120*, 209–212. https://doi.org/10.1016/j.paid.2017.09.006

Otu, A., Charles, C. H., & Yaya, S. (2020). Mental health and psychosocial well-being during the COVID-19 pandemic: The invisible elephant in the room. *International Journal of Mental Health Systems, 14*, 1–5. https://doi.org/10.1186/s13033-020-00371-w

Paredes, M. R., Apaolaza, V., Fernandez-Robin, C., Hartmann, P., & Yañez-Martinez, D. (2021). The impact of the COVID-19 pandemic on subjective mental well-being: The interplay of perceived threat, future anxiety and resilience. *Personality and Individual Differences, 170*, 110455. https://doi.org/10.1016/j.paid.2020.110455

Pennebaker, J. W., & Smyth, J. (2016). *Opening up by writing it down: How expressive writing improves health and eases emotional pain* (3rd ed.). Guilford Press.

Prime, H., Wade, M., & Browne, D. T. (2020). Risk and resilience in family well-being during the COVID-19 pandemic. *American Psychologist, 75*(5), 631–645. https://doi.org/10.1037/amp0000660

Puente-Martínez, A., Páez, D., Ubillos-Landa, S., & Da Costa-Dutra, S. (2018). Examining the structure of negative emotion regulation and its association with hedonic and psychological wellbeing. *Frontiers in Psychology, 9*. https://doi.org/10.3389/fpsyg.2018.01592

Restubog, S. L. D., Ocampo, A. C. G., & Wang, L. (2020). Taking control amidst the chaos: Emotion regulation during the COVID-19 pandemic. *Journal of Vocational Behaviour, 119* (June 2020), 103440. https://doi.org/10.1016/j.jvb.2020.103440

Shanahan, L., Steinhoff, A., Bechtiger, L., Murray, A. L., Nivette, A., Hepp, U., Ribeaud, D., & Eisner, M. (2020). Emotional distress in young adults during the COVID-19 pandemic: Evidence of risk and resilience from a longitudinal cohort study. *Psychological Medicine*, 1–10. https://doi.org/10.1017/S003329172000241X

Tee, E. Y. J., Raja Reza Shah, R. I. A., Thomas, K. S., Ng, S., & Phoo, E. Y. M. (2021, March 24). Beyond resilience: Promotive and protective traits that facilitate recovery during crisis. *PsyArXiv*. https://doi.org/10.31234/osf.io/p2h35

Thomas, C., & Zolkoski, S. (2020). Preventing stress among undergraduate learners: The importance of emotional intelligence, resilience, and emotion regulation. *Frontiers in Education, 5*, 1–8. https://doi.org/10.3389/feduc.2020.00094

Ungar, M., & Theron, L. (2020). Resilience and mental health: How multisystemic processes contribute to positive outcomes. *The Lancet Psychiatry, 7*(5), 441–448. https://doi.org/10.1016/S2215-0366(19)30434-1

Verzeletti, C., Zammuner, V. L., Galli, C., & Agnoli, S. (2016). Emotion regulation strategies and psychosocial well-being in adolescence. *Cogent Psychology, 3*(1). https://doi.org/10.1080/23311908.2016.1199294

Wong, L. P., Alias, H., Md Fuzi, A. A., Omar, I. S., Mohamad Nor, A., Tan, M. P., Baranovich, D. L., Saari, C. Z., Hamzah, S. H., Cheong, K. W., Poon, C. H., Ramoo, V., Che, C. C., Myint, K., Zainuddin, S., & Chung, I. (2021). Escalating progression of mental health disorders during the COVID-19 pandemic: Evidence from a nationwide survey. *PLoS ONE, 16*(3). https://doi.org/10.1371/journal.pone.0248916

World Health Organization (2004). Promoting mental health: Concepts, emerging evidence, practice. WHO.

Yunus, W. M. A. W. M., Badri, S. K. Z., Panatik, S. A., & Mukhtar, F. (2020). The unprecedented movement control order (lockdown) and factors associated with the negative emotional symptoms, happiness, and work-life balance of Malaysian university students during the Coronavirus disease (COVID-19) pandemic. *Frontiers in Psychiatry, 11*. https://doi.org/10.3389/fpsyt.2020.566221